THE COMPLETE BOOK OF
NATURAL
THERAPIES

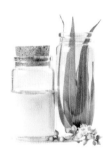

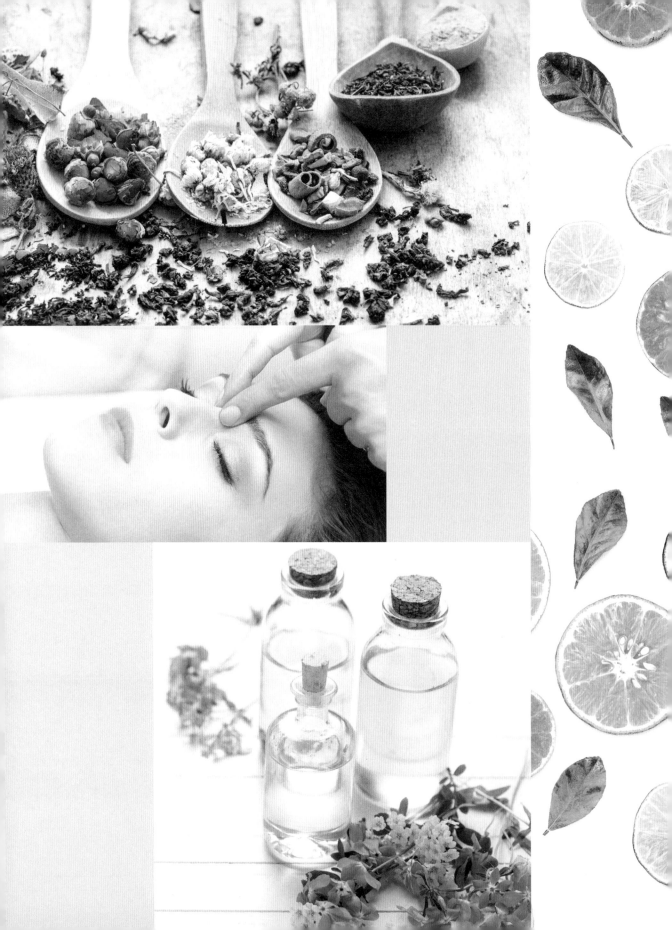

THE COMPLETE BOOK OF
NATURAL THERAPIES

SAFE AND EFFECTIVE SELF-HELP
FOR EVERYDAY AILMENTS

PETER ALBRIGHT, M.D.

METRO BOOKS
New York

METRO BOOKS
New York

An imprint of Sterling Publishing Co., Inc.
1166 Avenue of the Americas
New York, NY 10036

METRO BOOKS and the distinctive
Metro Books logo are registered
trademarks of Sterling Publishing Co., Inc.

Copyright © 1997 & 2019
Quarto Publishing plc,
an imprint of The Quarto Group

ISBN 978-1-4351-6831-2

For information about custom editions,
special sales, and premium and corporate
purchases, please contact Sterling Special
Sales at 800-805-5489 or specialsales@
sterlingpublishing.com.

2 4 6 8 10 9 7 5 3 1

sterlingpublishing.com

Conceived, edited, and designed by
Quarto Publishing plc
an imprint of The Quarto Group
The Old Brewery
6 Blundell Street
London N7 9BH
www.quartoknows.com

QUAR 304063

Editor: Michelle Pickering
Designers: Jackie Palmer, Michelle Pickering
Editorial assistant: Cassie Lawrence
Art director: Jess Hibbert
Publisher: Samantha Warrington

Printed in China

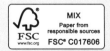

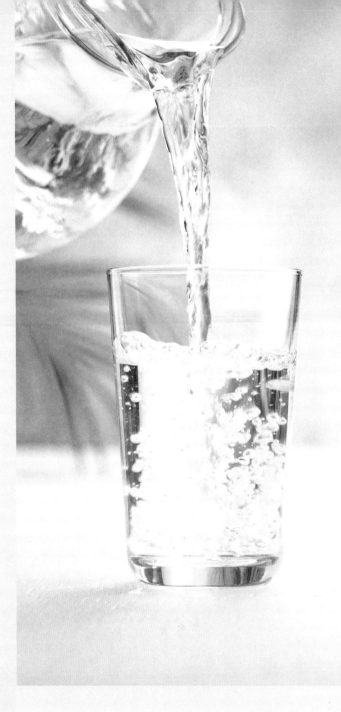

Publisher's note: This book is not intended as a
substitute for the advice of a health care professional.
The reader should regularly consult a health care
practitioner in matters relating to health, particularly
with respect to symptoms that may require diagnosis
or medical attention.

CONTENTS

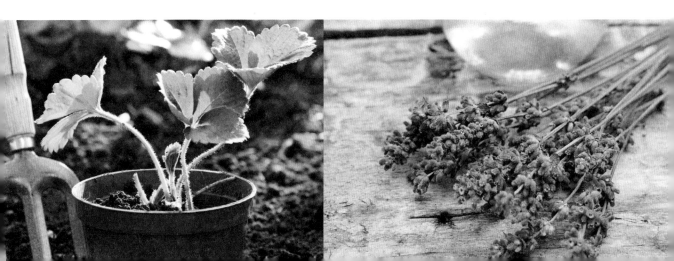

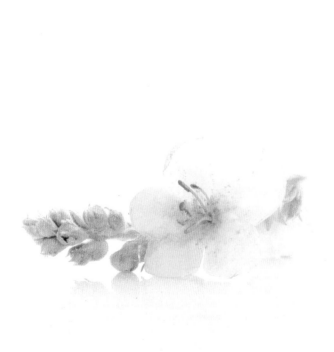
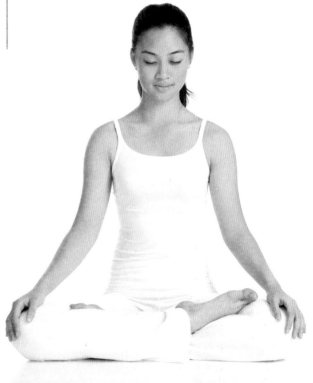

THERAPIES

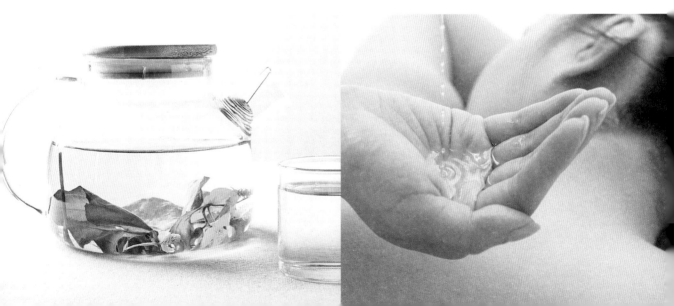

INTRODUCTION

This book is written to help the many millions of people frequently faced with health-related situations in their homes that are puzzling and perplexing. We are in the age of information explosion, but our biggest problem is how to filter out what information is useful to us from what is quite irrelevant. This book puts at your fingertips the information you will need when faced with any one of a hundred or so of the most common symptoms you are likely to encounter in yourself or in any member of your family.

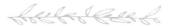

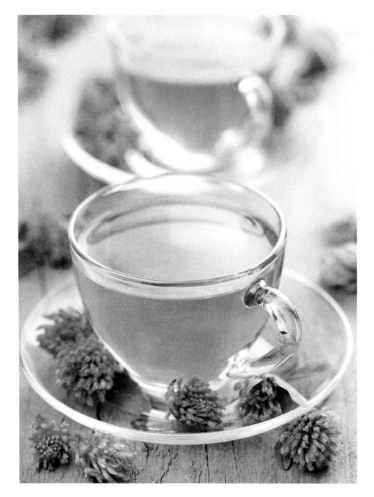

Although this is a book about symptoms of ill health and how to deal with them, it seems appropriate to put all this into the larger framework of wellness. The concept of wellness has grown to represent a state of being that is much more encompassing than just being momentarily healthy or between bouts of illness! The idea of wellness rests on the knowledge that we are complex beings in whom, from moment to moment, there is a subtle interaction among body, mind, emotions, and spirit, with all of them connecting to the environment in which we live and with the other beings who inhabit it.

Herbs such as red clover have a long history in the treatment of illness. One of the easiest ways to use herbal remedies is to drink them as infusions (teas).

How to Use This Book

First let us talk about how to use this book. It is really very simple—try it right now while you have it in your hand. Think of a symptom you would like to know more about—for example, headache. Turn to the contents page at the front of the book, where all the symptoms discussed are listed; then turn to the page indicated and you are in business!

There you will find a description of the most common types of headache, what events inside the body can give rise to a headache, how headaches are usually treated by a doctor, and how you can deal with headaches on your own. This includes a brief discussion of the complementary and alternative methods of managing a headache that are safe and effective. It also tells you how to decide whether the headache is too serious a problem for you to tackle and what to do if home management does not bring relief.

What do we mean by "complementary" and "alternative" methods? The first term refers to any form of treatment or management of a situation that complements what a doctor would do in the same situation, implying that a combination of the two might be more effective than either one used separately. This is different from "alternative" therapy, a term some people use to mean something you do instead of what the doctor might do. Many doctors now use both conventional and complementary methods to bring about relief of symptoms.

As the various complementary/alternative approaches are discussed, you will be referred to another section of the book, in which over 25 different therapies are discussed in more detail. This will help you to understand more about each one and how they might help you at home. In the case of headache, for example, you are referred only to the therapies that are known to be helpful for headache.

In the back of the book is advice on how to find a therapist or teacher who will help you to master a particular therapy so that you can use it with confidence in your own home.

SYMPTOMS

Associated symptoms

Conventional treatments list

Complementary therapies

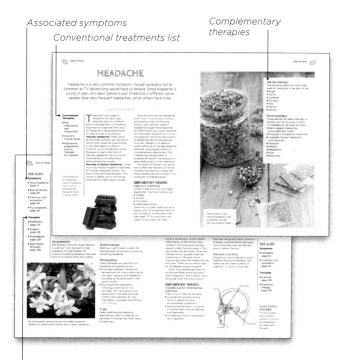

Cross-refers to additional therapies that may be useful

THERAPIES

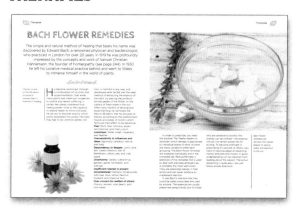

In-depth therapeutic solutions

A harvest of fresh fruits and vegetables along with seeds, nuts, and whole grains form the basis of a healthy diet.

A reflexologist treats various areas of the body through corresponding reflex points on the foot, stimulating energy to promote healing.

HOLISTIC MEDICINE

It is this understanding that lies behind the development of holistic medicine. The holistic concept sees each individual at the center of his or her universe. At any given moment, the individual is in connection with that universe in an infinite number of ways, including:

- through all of the events of that person's unique history
- through manifold personal interactions, past and present
- through many kinds of stresses, painful and pleasurable
- through a spiritual awareness, however difficult to define, and
- through a sense of direction along life's path.

Each new moment brings with it a slightly new perspective and new opportunities for the living of one's life. It also brings a subtle recombination of forces and new hope.

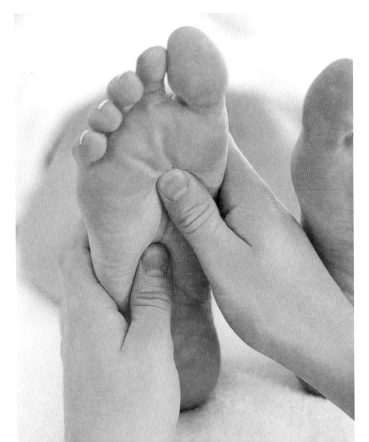

THE PURSUIT OF WELLNESS

Within this context we can think about what might be the most important things in our daily lives that can lead us toward this desirable state of wellness. I must emphasize the following areas in the pursuit of this goal.

Understanding and practicing good nutrition: This has long been recognized as of primary importance. In the past two or three decades, a great deal of new information has emerged that, combined with older wisdom, gives us a fresh look at the subject.

Using appropriate physical conditioning and exercise: Many people find this the easiest area to neglect or let slide in a program of wellness! It is not a matter of becoming a fitness addict, but rather of choosing the level of physical activity most appropriate to your circumstances and then practicing it consistently.

Seeking a true sense of vocation in one's work: This is a much neglected area in the study of the human condition. We often speak of the necessity of "jobs" being available in our culture, but the quality or suitability of such employment is seldom considered. Wherever possible it is important to view our life's work as a vocation, imbued with the highest sense of purpose of which we are capable.

Engaging in a daily practice of quietness or centering: This kind of meditative practice can put us in touch with our inner self and even our spiritual nature. It goes far beyond mere relaxation, although that is a wonderful by-product.

Developing healthy, open, and loving personal interactions: A very high percentage of our everyday stresses reside in this area, whether at home, at work, or elsewhere. We now know that turbulence in our emotional

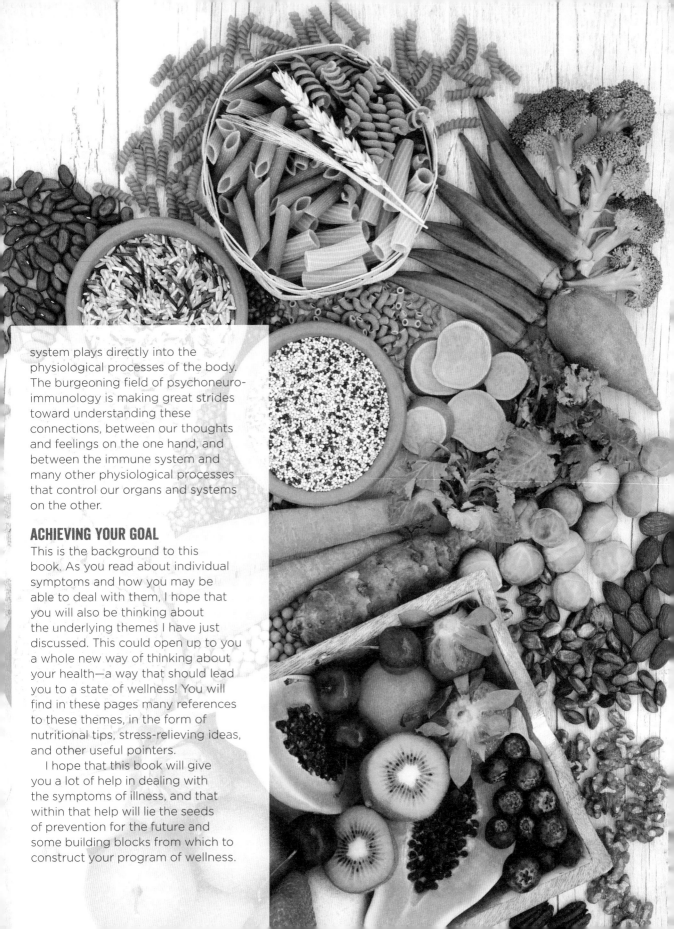

system plays directly into the physiological processes of the body. The burgeoning field of psychoneuro-immunology is making great strides toward understanding these connections, between our thoughts and feelings on the one hand, and between the immune system and many other physiological processes that control our organs and systems on the other.

ACHIEVING YOUR GOAL

This is the background to this book. As you read about individual symptoms and how you may be able to deal with them, I hope that you will also be thinking about the underlying themes I have just discussed. This could open up to you a whole new way of thinking about your health—a way that should lead you to a state of wellness! You will find in these pages many references to these themes, in the form of nutritional tips, stress-relieving ideas, and other useful pointers.

I hope that this book will give you a lot of help in dealing with the symptoms of illness, and that within that help will lie the seeds of prevention for the future and some building blocks from which to construct your program of wellness.

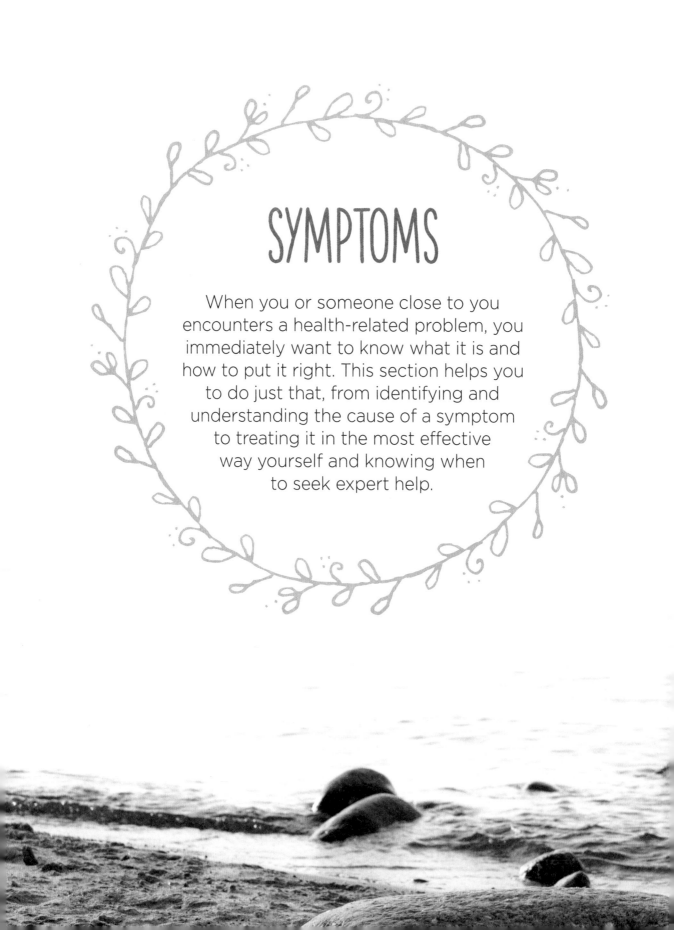

SYMPTOMS

When you or someone close to you encounters a health-related problem, you immediately want to know what it is and how to put it right. This section helps you to do just that, from identifying and understanding the cause of a symptom to treating it in the most effective way yourself and knowing when to seek expert help.

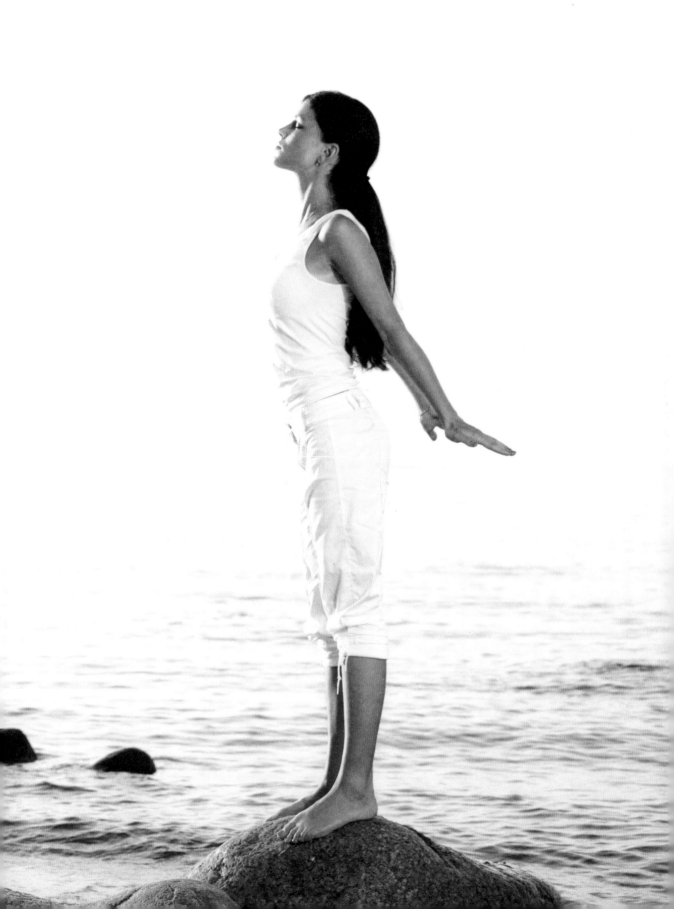

FIRST AID FOR PAIN

Many of the treatments and remedies in this section are to be found later in this book, but are summarized here for quick reference in an emergency. The treatments and remedies covered are for adults but may also be safely used (unless stated otherwise) for babies and children. Where medicines are concerned, use half the adult quantity or less, according to the instructions on the bottle or package.

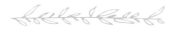

A purpose-made gelatin cold pack is a quick and effective remedy for both bruises and sprains.

Everyone experiences unexpected injuries and illnesses at one time or another, and quick treatment may be essential both to alleviate pain and to prevent the problem from escalating.

BRUISES

Place anything cold on the affected part as soon as possible, and leave for about 10–15 minutes. An ice pack, a bag of frozen peas from the freezer, or simply a washcloth soaked in cold water will do.

Arnica is the best remedy for mild to moderate bruising, and hypericum for severe bruising. Apply either as a cream over the entire area after icing and drying the bruise. The homeopathic remedy arnica 6c will also help, or if the bones under the bruise feel sore, symphytum 6c (alternatives are ruta and bellis per). For a black eye, lachesis 6c is best. In all cases, take one tablet every hour for four hours.

Alternatives to arnica are comfrey cream and aloe vera gel. A cold compress soaked in tincture of comfrey can also be beneficial.

SPRAINS

As for bruises, place an ice pack or similar on the affected part, and keep it there for as long as possible.

Immerse the sprain for about 15 minutes in a bowl of cold water containing four drops of the essential oils of rosemary and sweet marjoram. Make a cold compress using the same liquid, wrap it around the sprain, and keep it in place (using a waterproof bandage or similar) for several hours.

Take the homeopathic remedies arnica 6c (every half hour for two hours) and ruta 6c (three times a day for a week).

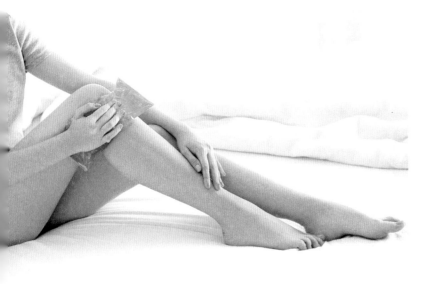

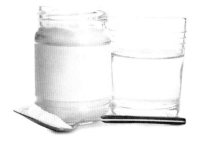

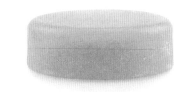

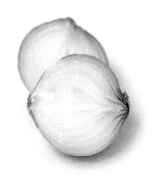

CUTS

Clean the cut with warm water and flush with calendula tincture (or apply calendula ointment). If the cut is deep, apply firm pressure for several minutes after cleaning to help stop the bleeding, preferably using a lint or cotton pad. Check that there is no loss of sensation or impeded function. Protect with a sterile pad, clean handkerchief, adhesive tape, or bandage.

Hypericum 6c helps to promote healing and overcome shock. Take a pill every hour for four hours.

BITES

Bites from any creature, animal or human can be serious if deep enough, and infection is always a risk. So, in addition to washing and cleaning the wound, and applying an antiseptic (tea tree oil is excellent), always seek medical help as soon as possible. This step is essential if the bite is from a wild animal, snake, or dog. For minor bites, the homeopathic remedies hypericum, apis, and staphysagria may help reduce any swelling and pain.

STINGS

Calamine lotion is a good general remedy for minor stings, but not for stings from bees and wasps.

Insect stings: The homeopathic remedy ledum 6c is good for all stings, but particularly those where the skin has been punctured, relieving pain and swelling. Calendula cream and witch hazel tincture can also reduce swelling and soothe pain. The homeopathic tincture pyrethrum and Bach Rescue Remedy may also help.

Bee stings: Sodium bicarbonate will neutralize the poison. Dissolve two teaspoonfuls in a cup of warm water and apply with a cotton ball. Apis 12c (one tablet every half hour until the pain stops) is effective for both bee and wasp stings.

Wasp stings: Vinegar or lemon juice, applied to the skin undiluted, will neutralize the poison.

Jellyfish stings: A hot bath is the best way to neutralize the poison in jellyfish stings. The temperature should be 100–102°F (38–39°C). For severe stings, take the homeopathic remedy apis 30c (take one tablet every hour until the stinging stops). Ledum and calendula can also be beneficial.

Nettle stings: Rubbing a dock leaf onto the affected area is very effective (docks are usually found where nettles grow). The leaf should be rubbed on vigorously, so that the juice from the leaf goes into the skin to neutralize the poison.

Poison ivy stings: Cut an onion in half and rub it on the affected area. Wash the area with soap and water to remove the plant's oil, and apply a paste of sodium bicarbonate and water as for bee stings.

CAUTION

Reactions to some stings, notably from insects (especially bees and wasps) and jellyfish, can sometimes be so severe as to be life-threatening. This kind of allergic reaction is known as anaphylaxis. Signs are cold, clammy skin with an itchy rash, rapid, shallow breathing, and weak pulse. Seek immediate medical help.

To treat poison ivy stings, rub a cut onion on the affected area, then wash with soap and water, and follow with an application of sodium bicarbonate paste.

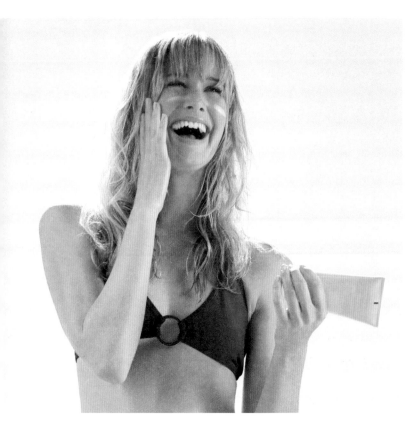

Too much sun is dangerous and the use of sun block is essential, especially in fair-skinned people.

SUNBURN

Soak for 15–20 minutes in a tub of cold water mixed with one of the following: several drops of lavender oil or vinegar, or a sprinkling of sodium bicarbonate or oatmeal.

Dry and gently rub in either aloe vera gel, vitamin E cream, or calendula ointment. A cold compress of calendula tincture, held in place, can help soothe badly affected areas. Sunburned eyelids benefit from a slice of fresh cucumber left on them for at least 15 minutes.

SUNSTROKE

Sunstroke (or heatstroke) is characterized by a splitting headache, neck pain, feverishness, dizziness, nausea, and a rapid pulse. The immediate aim is to bring down the body temperature, so sit in a cold bathtub or wrap the body in a sheet soaked in cold water. Seek immediate medical help if body temperature has not dropped after about an hour.

These homeopathic remedies may help: belladonna 6c (for a high temperature), glonoin 6c (for dizziness), and cuprum 6c (for cramp).

CAUTION
Too much sun can be extremely dangerous, especially for children and light-skinned people. Severe sunburn and sunstroke can be life-threatening. If in doubt, seek immediate medical help.

CHILBLAINS

Twice a day put the affected hands or feet into hot water for two minutes, then cold water for one minute. Repeat five times. If the affected parts are bleeding, apply calendula cream after the bathing. If they are not bleeding, apply arnica tincture diluted in cold water (six drops to a pint/570ml). Soak a washcloth in the mixture, wring out, and leave on overnight.

BURNS AND SCALDS

For minor burns and scalds, place the affected part under cool running water for at least 10 minutes. Mix 10 drops of hypericum tincture in a glass of cold water and pour over. Dry and cover with a clean, sterile dressing. Bach Rescue Remedy may help any after-effects. For severe pain, one tablet of the homeopathic remedy aconite 12c may bring relief.

Alternatively, place an ice pack on the burn or scald for 10 minutes, then apply aloe vera tincture or calendula ointment. Or, soak some gauze in witch hazel and bandage it carefully onto the affected area.

CAUTION
Severe burns or scalds, especially those covering large areas, can produce life-threatening traumatic shock, and require immediate medical attention.

FROSTBITE

Remove anything covering the affected area and warm it slowly between the hands. Do not rub the skin. Dab on Friar's balsam or tincture of myrrh and loosely cover with a dry dressing. Wrap in a blanket to keep warm, and wear gloves and socks. Take agaricus 12c immediately, apis 6c if there is swelling, and pulsatilla 6c if heat makes the condition worse. Take a high-potency vitamin B-complex capsule and 400 iu of vitamin E daily.

CAUTION

Frostbite is a serious condition, and immediate medical help is necessary.

NAUSEA AND VOMITING

For all forms of nausea and vomiting, including travel or motion sickness (car, air, and sea sickness) and morning sickness during pregnancy, take ginger. Make it into a tea (cut the root into pieces, simmer for about 15 minutes, and drink); or take it in capsules (two half an hour before traveling, or as necessary for other forms of nausea); or simply chew the raw root. Eating crystallized ginger during a journey can also be effective.

The herbs Roman chamomile and black horehound can also reduce nausea and vomiting, but do NOT take if pregnant.

Take the homeopathic remedies nux vomica together with cocculus (both 6c) for general nausea and vomiting; sepia 6c for nausea brought on by the smell of food; pulsatilla, ipecacuanha, arsenicum album (all 6c) for motion sickness; tabacum 6c if symptoms include sweating and giddiness; and borax 6c if there is anxiety.

Essential oil of peppermint can also help. Add four drops to a neutral oil, such as grapeseed, and rub onto the chest to be inhaled. Alternatively, put the drops onto a tissue or handkerchief and breathe in the vapor that way. Elasticized bands with a sewn-in acupressure stud, which can be worn on the wrist during a journey to help keep sickness at bay, are available from many drugstores and health food stores.

For motion sickness, if you do not have an acupressure wristband, press a point on the wrist in line with the largest (middle) finger, three fingers' width from the wrist crease nearest the hand for several seconds.

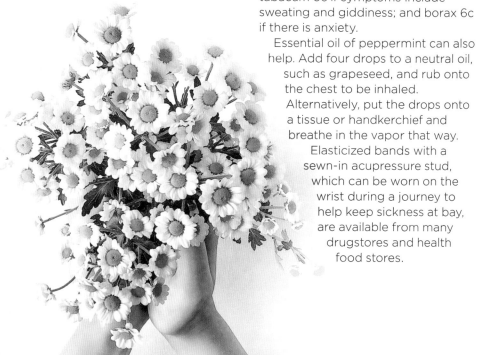

Roman camomile is often used for treating nausea and vomiting in cases such as motion sickness.

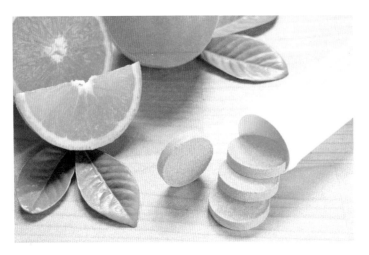

Effervescent vitamin C in water before sleep can help avoid hangover.

CRAMP

Press hard into the center of the painful area with the thumbs and try to stretch the muscle at the same time. While the cramp is easing, apply a hot compress—a washcloth soaked in hot water and wrung out will do. Repeat the application four or five times, then try gently working the muscle by stretching and kneading it.

Effective herbal remedies are kelp, ginko biloba, and crampbark (taken as tea), and the homeopathic cuprum 3c.

Eating plenty of dark green leafy vegetables together with shellfish, nuts, and seeds can help prevent attacks, as can daily supplementing with evening primrose or starflower (borage) oil (1g a day), vitamin C (3g), vitamin E (250–400 iu), calcium, and magnesium.

NOTE In hot countries, heavy sweating can cause cramp through loss of salt. Too much salt loss can lead to coma, so eat more salt with food. Magnesium supplements (500mg a day) may be necessary too.

HANGOVER

Drink at least a pint (570ml) of water with 1g of vitamin C before going to sleep, and peppermint, nettle, chamomile, or yarrow tea throughout the following day. Honey (12 teaspoonfuls), alone or in warm water, may also help.

TOOTHACHE

Apply oil of cloves to the sore area. Chewing a dried clove will achieve the same effect by releasing the anesthetic that the herb contains.

Homeopathic First Aid

For	Remedy	Dose
Severe pain (after injury)	Aconite	1 x 6c pill
Insect bites and stings	Apis	1 x 30c pill every half hour
Accidents or injuries	Arnica	1 x 6c pill every half hour
Bruises	Arnica	1–2 x 3c pills every half hour
Burns, blisters, scalds	Cantharis	1 x 6c pill
Anxiety and general pain relief	Chamomilla	1 x 30c pill as needed
Cuts and wounds	Hypericum	1 x 30c pill every hour for 3–4 hours
Hangover, motion sickness	Nux vomica	1 x 6c pill
Nosebleed from injury	Phosphate	1 x 6c pill
Muscular pain	Rhus tox	1 x 6c pill every hour

For best effect homeopathic pills should not be swallowed, but allowed to dissolve slowly under the tongue.

CHRONIC PAIN

Although pain is a feature of many of the conditions in this book, chronic, unremitting pain deserves separate consideration because it must be managed in different ways from acute pain. Often it must be considered apart from whatever condition is causing the pain.

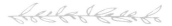

Pain sensations are carried as nerve impulses in the sensory components of the peripheral nerves serving all parts of the body. The interpretation of these nerve impulses takes place in the brain. Thus the intensity of pain can be influenced either at the peripheral end of the nerve or at the site of interpretation in the brain. Soothing ointments work at the periphery, pain-relieving drugs in the brain. The threshold above which pain is appreciated by the brain varies significantly from person to person. It is also clear that the brain can be distracted by various activities, with partial or complete disappearance of pain for at least the duration of the distraction.

Another important concept involves natural substances in the body that have been called endorphins because of their ability to reduce pain, similar to the action of morphine (endomorphin). This phenomenon has been studied extensively, and it has been found that many things can influence endorphin levels in the body, including exercise, biofeedback, and imagery, with concomitant relief of pain.

Conventional Therapies

- Pain-relievers
- Surgery
- Pain clinics
- TENS devices (transcutaneous electrical nerve stimulation)

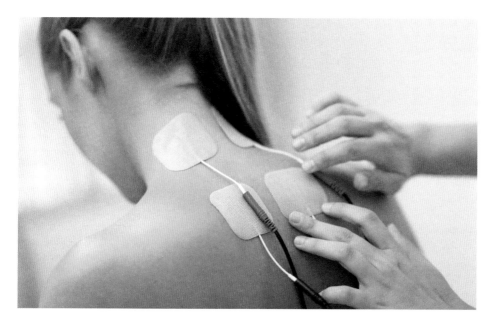

TENS devices applied to the skin have been found effective in many cases of chronic pain. The unit stimulates a nerve with a low-grade electric current, producing an effect that competes with pain perception taking place in the brain.

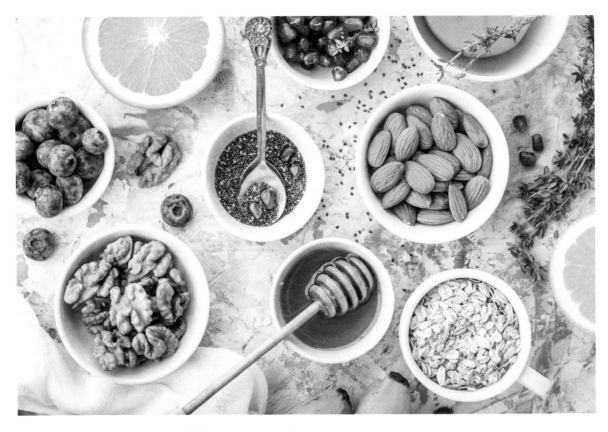

A healthy diet is important for maintaining good health and well-being.

COMPLEMENTARY THERAPIES
Diet and nutrition

In the face of chronic pain, for various reasons, diet patterns change and may become quite unbalanced, yet it is of paramount importance to maintain an optimal nutrition program. Just the stress of the illness or injury, plus the pain component, depletes the levels of vitamins and other nutrients in the body significantly. Melatonin, among its many virtues, enhances beta-endorphin activity.

Group therapy

An excellent example of group therapy is the modern pain clinic. A painful injury or other condition may leave a lasting legacy of pain long after the original physical injury has healed—phantom limb pain after an amputation is but one example. For this and other reasons, treatment facilities have come into being whose main purpose is to deal with the problem of chronic pain. These pain clinics are one of the best examples to be found in mainstream medicine of a multi-factorial or holistic approach to a health problem. A wide variety of approaches are integrated into a single therapeutic effort. These include physical therapy and conditioning, biofeedback, hypnosis, imagery, psychotherapy, occupational therapy, and social and family counseling. The results of such combined therapy have been very good in a high proportion of cases.

Biofeedback

Biofeedback has been found effective in controlling many types of pain. Learn the method first from a qualified trainer. Once you have bought a small amount of equipment, you can use the method in your home for as long as necessary.

Exercise

Exercise is effective in reducing the perception of pain by producing distraction and probably by other mechanisms as well. However, it must be tailored to any limitations imposed by the concomitant condition.

Acupressure

Acupressure has been found effective in low back and other pain. Acupuncture, while not a home therapy, is very effective in control of pain in the head, neck, shoulder, and arm areas.

Herbal therapy

- Arnica
- Bromelain
- Capsaicin
- Ginger
- Hypericum
- Sarapin

Imagery

Many investigators have found that imagery and self-hypnosis techniques are effective in reducing pain. It is necessary to learn such a method, preferably from a qualified teacher. Once learned, it can be used in the home indefinitely.

Meditation

The ability to go within to the place of quiet and calm has a beneficial effect in the management of pain. It is all the more useful if one has become familiar with the pathway before pain must be dealt with.

Yoga

The practice of hatha yoga, stressing mindfulness, meditation, and awareness of breathing, has been found to be helpful over time in reducing pain in various areas.

SEE ALSO

Symptoms

- Since chronic pain can be associated with many regions and systems in the body, you may wish to consult any other entry in the Symptoms section.

Therapies

- Alexander technique page 185
- Massage page 186
- Reflexology page 195
- Therapeutic touch page 212
- Stress management page 220
- Group therapy page 223
- Music therapy page 224
- Aromatherapy page 232
- Homeopathy page 244

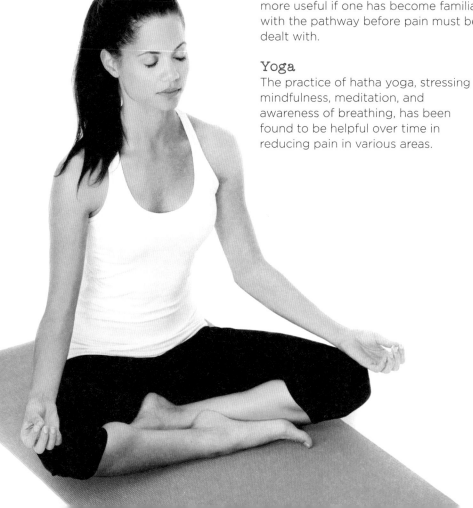

One of the most famous postures of hatha yoga: the lotus position.

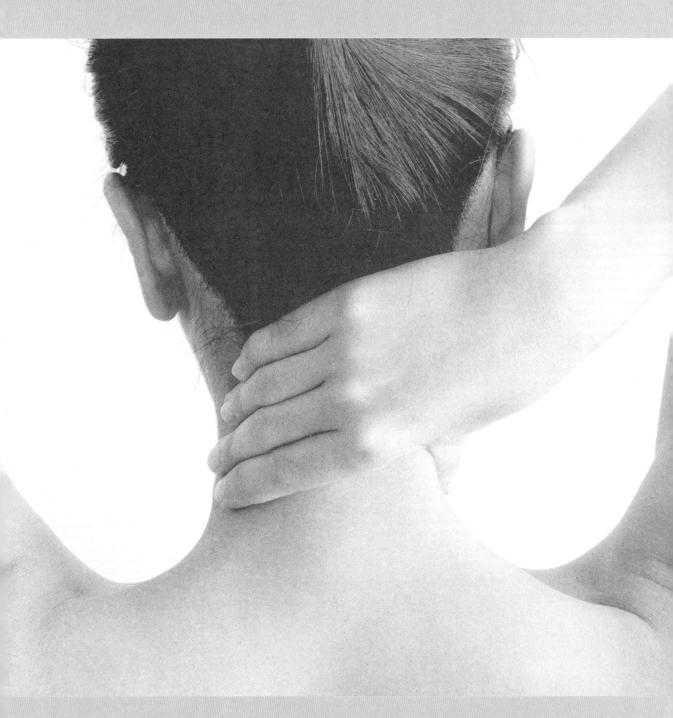

HEAD & NECK

HEADACHE

Headache is a very common symptom, though probably not as common as TV advertising would have us believe. Since headache is a kind of pain, and each person's pain threshold is different, some people have very frequent headaches, while others have none.

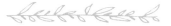

Conventional Therapies

- Pain medications and tranquilizers

- Over-the-counter drugs

- Ergotamine preparations, such as Cafergot, for migraine

Food sensitivity is a well-known cause of headache. Foods such as chocolate are frequently found to be the culprit.

There are many types of headache and each type responds best to a different kind of management. It is therefore important to diagnose which kind of headache is being experienced in order to treat it successfully.

Vascular headaches: These are by far the most common and are due to factors that cause the small arteries in the head region to dilate or constrict, i.e. to change their caliber. Migraine is a particular form of vascular headache, with distinctive characteristics, including visual disturbances and nausea.

Muscular or tension headaches: These occur as a result of spasm or tightness of muscles, especially those in the back of the neck and shoulders. This causes a steady pull on the tissues covering the scalp, producing pain.

Vascular and muscular headaches often occur in combination and are produced by many of the same factors. Less common types of headache include those produced by inflammation, as in sinus headache and meningitis; pressure, as in tumor; and eyestrain. Since the vast majority of headaches fall into the vascular/muscular category, it is safe and usually effective to manage headache episodes using a great variety of complementary approaches. Only if headaches are persistent or progressive should it be necessary to seek medical help in their treatment.

The object of therapy is to reduce the number and frequency of nerve impulses reaching the muscles and blood vessels that are involved in the production of headache pain.

COMPLEMENTARY THERAPIES
Diet and nutrition

Certain foods are known to trigger headaches. The most common are:
- Cheese
- Alcohol
- Chocolate
- Caffeinated drinks

Sensitivity to other foods may be to blame, and it is sometimes useful to put yourself on an elimination diet (see page 177) to track down the culprit in your particular case.

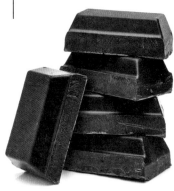

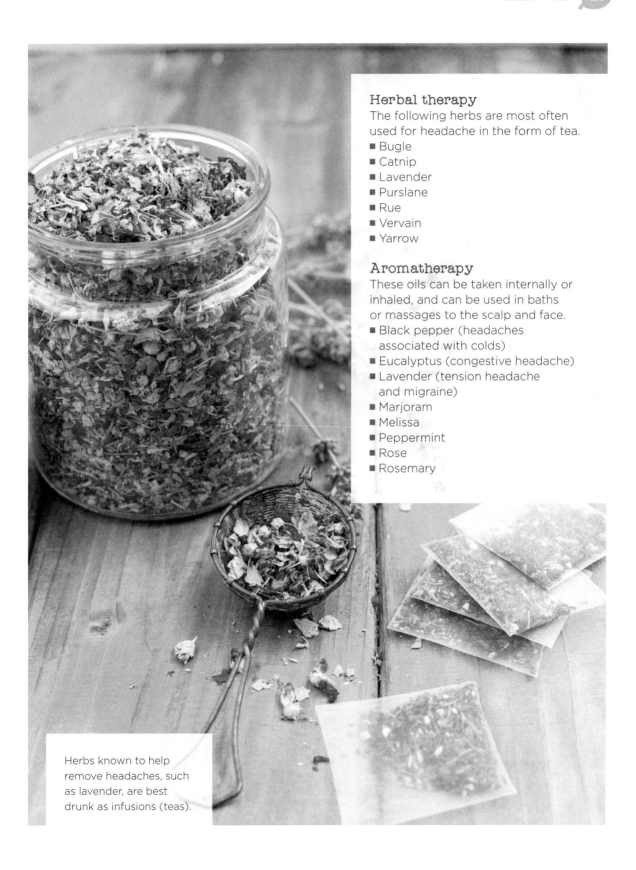

Herbal therapy

The following herbs are most often used for headache in the form of tea.

- Bugle
- Catnip
- Lavender
- Purslane
- Rue
- Vervain
- Yarrow

Aromatherapy

These oils can be taken internally or inhaled, and can be used in baths or massages to the scalp and face.

- Black pepper (headaches associated with colds)
- Eucalyptus (congestive headache)
- Lavender (tension headache and migraine)
- Marjoram
- Melissa
- Peppermint
- Rose
- Rosemary

Herbs known to help remove headaches, such as lavender, are best drunk as infusions (teas).

SEE ALSO

Symptoms

- Sinus headache
  page 27
- Eye symptoms
  page 28
- Common cold
  symptoms
  page 46
- Flu symptoms
  page 48

Therapies

- Meditation
  page 215
- Imagery
  page 218
- Biofeedback
  page 228
- Bach flower
  remedies
  page 236

Stress management

Check your stress patterns. Stress is implicated in most vascular headaches. There is a long list of stresses that you can check out and do something about. The most common and important are interpersonal relations, job stresses, and environmental factors, such as allergens, smog, foods, etc.

Exercise

Take up walking as a regular activity. This is the simplest and safest form of effective exercise. Find places near your home that are away from traffic and give you a sense of peace, traveling to them by car if necessary, in which to go walking. Your body and spirit will appreciate the change of scene and pace.

Acupressure

Gall bladder 14 and 20, large intestine 4, and liver 3 can be used to treat headache. For gall bladder 20, pressure should be applied at the level of C1-2, 1in (2.5cm) from the midline.

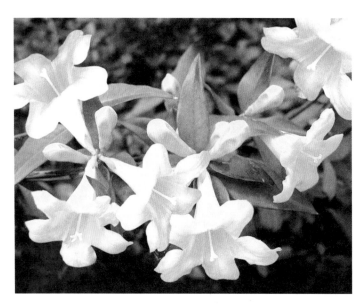

The homeopathic remedy derived from yellow jessamine (*Gelsemium sempervirens*) can be used to relieve headaches.

Massage

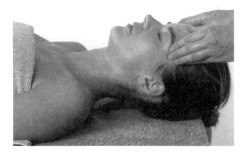

Self-massage of the neck and shoulder muscles can be very helpful. Massage is even more beneficial if administered by a caring friend. Light, sensitive pressure to the temples with the fingertips can induce fast relief from headaches. A soft, circular motion eases muscle tension, relaxing nerves and encouraging emotional release.

Hydrotherapy

Bathing in warm water is useful for relaxing away the tension so prone to producing headache.

Homeopathy

These remedies are used both for headache and general tension.

- Focusing ingredient: Gelsemium sempervirens 4x—this is effective for neuralgia, migraine, and headaches provoked by displacements in the spinal column.
- Accompanying ingredients: Cimicifuga racemosa 4x—for neuralgia, cervical migraine, and severe pain in the head and eyes; or Rhus toxicodexdron 4x—for rheumatism, neuralgia, and stiffness upon moving.

Yoga

Deep breathing and relaxation exercises are useful in relieving the tightness in muscles that often leads to head pain.

SINUS HEADACHE

Sinus headache is a specific head pain often incorrectly diagnosed by the sufferer. In many cases self-described as sinus headache, no sinus inflammation is present and the headache is actually a symptom of the common cold. However, sinusitis can be a sequel to a cold.

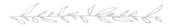

The true sinus headache occurs as a result of sinus inflammation, which blocks the tiny passage between a sinus and the nasal cavity. This causes pressure within the sinus and produces the pain.

A reliable sign that can be noted at home is tenderness. When there is inflammation of the frontal sinus, located in the brow area, pressing upward under the bony edge of the eye socket may elicit pain. When the maxillary sinus, located inside the cheekbone, is inflamed, thumb pressure up under the cheekbone may elicit pain. There are no similiar signs for the deeper sinuses, however.

Other, more generalized signs of sinusitis are fever, aches and pains, nasal congestion, and a yellow, sticky discharge when the nose is blown.

COMPLEMENTARY THERAPIES
Combating environmental pollution
There is much that can be done.
- Consider the location of your home in relation to local environmental conditions.
- Avoid airborne toxins, if possible, or control them with air cleaners and fresheners.
- Humidifying the air is sometimes very important.

Herbal therapy
- Bee propolis
- Echinacea
- Garlic
- Goldenseal

Hydrotherapy
Use nasal lavage and steam inhalation to loosen nasal secretions and apply cold compresses over the affected sinus to relieve the pain.

Diet and nutrition
Choose your food carefully to avoid ingesting toxins and allergens, and make sure that there is plenty of vitamins C, A, and E in your diet.

Conventional Therapies
- Antibiotics
- Decongestants
- Pain-relievers

SEE ALSO
Symptoms
- Headache page 24
- Common cold symptoms page 46

Therapies
- Exercise page 180
- Breathing therapy page 190

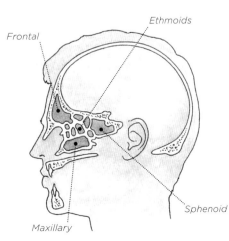

Frontal

Ethmoids

Sphenoid

Maxillary

PARANASAL SINUSES
The four sinuses are air cavities located in the brow, the cheekbones, and deep within the skull.

EYE SYMPTOMS

It is generally acknowledged, by eye doctors and lay persons alike, that the eye is a vitally important organ and that its integrity is to be preserved at all costs. All efforts will be bent in that direction when there is a question about vision. The first resort whenever eye symptoms arise should be to consult an eye doctor.

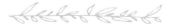

Conventional Therapies

- Topical antibiotics
- Steroids
- Surgery

Once the doctor has established that there is no eye disease present and that lens correction is not required, then you may safely consider what courses are open to you for handling the symptoms. Also, if it is not an emergency situation, you might have to wait for an appointment to see an eye doctor, so you may want to think about certain symptoms and their possible meanings.

Pain in the eye: By itself, pain may signify an increase in pressure inside the eye, or simply eyestrain. If you do not wear glasses, check to see if the eye pain comes toward the end of the working day—if so, you may need glasses. In the meantime, rest your eyes for a few minutes and that may ease the pain temporarily. If pain in the eye is accompanied by blurring or reduced vision, you had better see a doctor right away. Pain in one eye or the eyebrow region, sometimes with blurring or flashing in the eye, may signify a "migraine equivalent." A doctor can confirm such a diagnosis, which will be treated differently from an eye problem.

Blurring of vision: Several conditions produce blurring. A common—and benign—one is called floaters. These are small aggregates of cells that float around inside the eye. They are very noticeable when they occur, but one gets used to them in time, so that they are mostly invisible. Another common cause of blurring is cataracts, a condition where the lens of the eye develops a cloudy spot that grows and interferes with vision. Many people with a cataract have surgery, which is now comparatively simple. Other conditions in the eye can cause blurring—usually an eye doctor's skill is required to diagnose them.

Double vision: This can be due to a simple refractive error, but it can also be an indication of some problem with the nerves and muscles that move the eyeball. In either case, it is a good idea to have an eye examination, unless the symptom is only very slight and goes away with resting the eyes.

Visual loss: Loss of vision can mean a number of things, with parts of the visual fields of one or both eyes being affected. They all require a thorough examination by an eye doctor to sort them out and indicate treatment.

"Have your eyesight tested regularly and consult an eye doctor about any problems before you treat them."

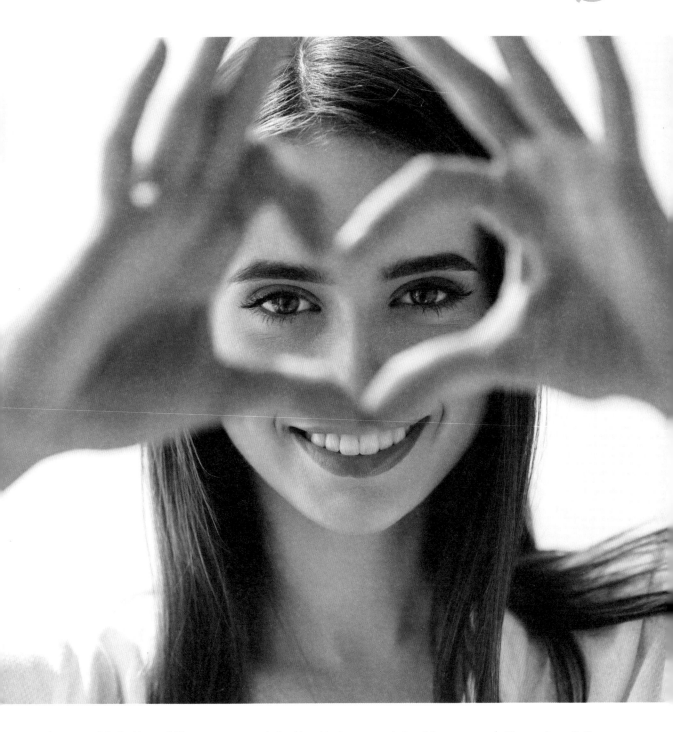

Redness and irritation of the eyes: The commonest cause is environmental—the irritants in the air around us. The next commonest is conjunctivitis, a simple bacterial infection that responds best to antibiotic eye ointments. To prevent these things, we need to examine our lifestyle carefully.

The eye is a vitally important organ, so it is essential to take good care of your eye health.

SEE ALSO

Symptoms

- Common cold symptoms page 46
- Diabetic symptoms page 158
- Symptoms relating to immune function page 166
- Aging page 170

Therapies

- Biofeedback page 228
- Homeopathy page 244

COMPLEMENTARY THERAPIES

Herbal therapy

- Borage
- Calendula
- Carrot
- Chamomile
- Chickweed
- Cucumber
- Dandelion
- Elderflower
- Goldenseal
- Marigold
- Red eyebright

Bates method

This is a method in which exercises are performed daily to strengthen the muscles of the eye. It has been found to be effective by many, instead of or in addition to glasses. The method may be useful in cases where eyestrain or eye inflammation is prominent.

Acupressure

Use gall bladder 20, stomach 3, and large intestine 4 to relieve eye symptoms. Large intestine 4 is especially useful for eye infections, but do not apply pressure here during pregnancy.

Hydrotherapy

This is useful for giving quick relief from eyestrain without the need for special ingredients. Simply place a dampened towel over your eyes, alternating between cold and warm towels.

Combating environmental pollution

Air pollution is a major problem in urban society and a major cause of eye irritation. It may be a significant factor in deciding where to live. You may find that air cleaners provide relief in the home, but in severe cases, more drastic measures, such as moving to a less polluted area, may be the only answer. We must all actively support measures to reduce air pollution.

Diet and nutrition

Cod liver oil has been used safely and effectively to prevent a rise in intraocular pressure in early or borderline glaucoma, which is a form of eye disease. Take one to two teaspoons daily.

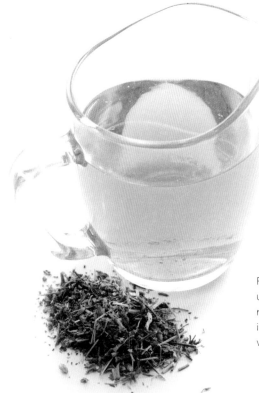

For eyestrain, bathe the eye with euphrasia, either using an eye-cup (eye-bath) or by soaking some roll cotton (cotton wool) in the liquid and applying it to your eye for around 20 minutes every hour while the pain lasts.

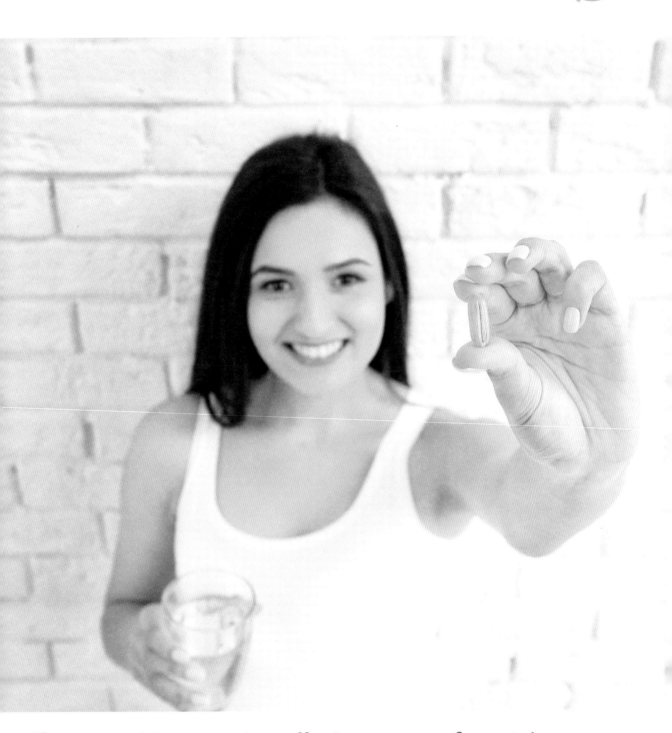

"Cod liver oil has proved an effective treatment for certain symptoms of eye pressure. Rich in vitamins A and D, it can also be taken in capsules to avoid the problem of its fishy odor."

EARACHE AND EAR DISCHARGE

Earache is still a common affliction in children and almost always denotes inflammation or infection in the middle ear (otitis media), which is often a complication of tonsillitis.

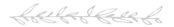

Conventional Therapies

- Antibiotics
- Decongestants
- Pain-relievers
- Insertion of plastic tubes through the eardrum to relieve pressure

Otitis media, a bacterial or viral infection, causes inflammatory blocking of the eustachean tube connecting the ear to the throat. This produces a buildup of pressure in the middle ear, with considerable pain. Children who are susceptible to this condition tend to have less trouble as they get older, as the passages are more spacious and less prone to blockage.

Discharge from the external ear is usually the result of infection there, except when tubes are in place for the treatment of otitis media.

COMPLEMENTARY THERAPIES

Diet and nutrition

Milk and other dairy products appear to predispose children to otitis media and other upper respiratory infections. Eliminating or reducing fats, cholesterol, wheat, dairy products, and sugar is effective. The addition of adequate nutrient supplementation is essential in childhood because of the many stresses encountered, the most important of which is growth itself.

Herbal therapy

The following herbs are used mostly in the form of gargles to treat ear and throat problems.
- Echinacea
- Goldenseal
- Mullein
- Peppermint
- Slippery elm
- Tansy

Hydrotherapy

- Inhalation of steam, with or without tincture of benzoin, works to relieve inflammation and blockage.
- Hot baths of short duration are relaxing and stimulate circulation to the affected part.

Aromatherapy

- Basil, chamomile, hyssop, lavender, savory, and rose
- Cajuput (inflammation)

STRUCTURE OF THE EAR

Ear problems can affect the ear canals, the middle ear, and the eustachean tube to the throat.

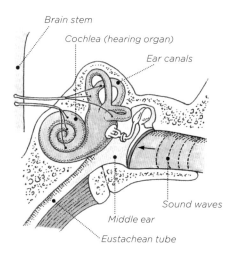

Brain stem

Cochlea (hearing organ)

Ear canals

Sound waves

Middle ear

Eustachean tube

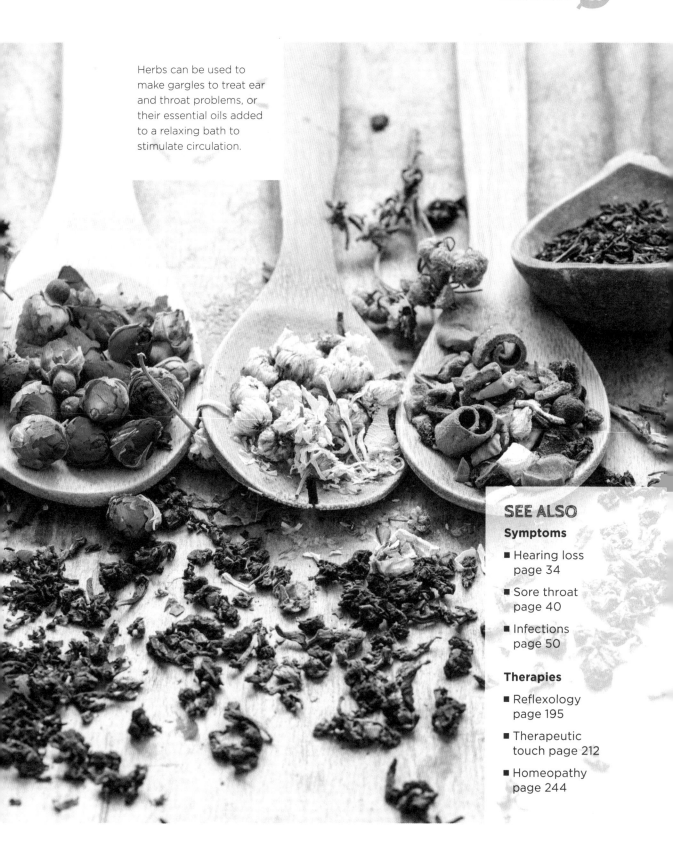

Herbs can be used to make gargles to treat ear and throat problems, or their essential oils added to a relaxing bath to stimulate circulation.

SEE ALSO

Symptoms

- Hearing loss page 34

- Sore throat page 40

- Infections page 50

Therapies

- Reflexology page 195

- Therapeutic touch page 212

- Homeopathy page 244

HEARING LOSS

Hearing loss may be divided into acute and chronic types. The latter is one of the most insidious of problems—a subtle, gradual, and subjective alteration of reality, often denied for a long time by the sufferer but noticed by others. Eventually it reaches the point where the subject is so inconvenienced by it that something must be done.

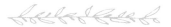

Conventional Therapies

- Antibiotics for acute and chronic infections
- Manual removal of wax or other obstruction
- Surgery

Meditation can help those suffering from hearing loss to feel more connected with the world around them.

An examination by a competent audiologist is a good first step. This will detect whether the problem is caused by wax accumulation, and if not, will determine the type of deafness and see if it can be corrected to a reasonable degree. We often see people who cannot get adequate correction, who gradually drift off into their own world. These people should be encouraged to take the initiative and to try some other way of

Prevention

A widely neglected practice is the use of hearing protection in situations where loud noise could cause damage. Excessively loud music has complicated this situation in recent years, as has the use of a variety of power tools. We need to be aware of those situations in which we might sustain permanent damage, either from short peaks of noise (e.g. gunshot) or sustained sound (e.g. a chain saw). The alternative may be irreversible loss of hearing.

compensating, such as lipreading or sign language. It involves calling more attention to the disability, but it is worth it to maintain a connection with the rest of the world.

Among the causes of chronic hearing loss is a familial type called otosclerosis, in which the tiny bony ossicles of the middle ear become fused, losing their ability to vibrate in response to sound waves. This can only be diagnosed accurately by a professional examination or an audiogram. Once diagnosed, the situation can be improved by an operation called a stapedectomy.

COMPLEMENTARY THERAPIES
Meditation

Perhaps the most useful thing you can do on your own is to try to get in touch with your inner calmness and confidence in order to help you feel less cut off from the world and to focus more on friends and family. Then you will have the incentive to take other steps to enhance your connections with people.

Herbal therapy

- Echinacea
- Ginkgo biloba
- Goldenseal
- Tinctures of warm mullein flower oil

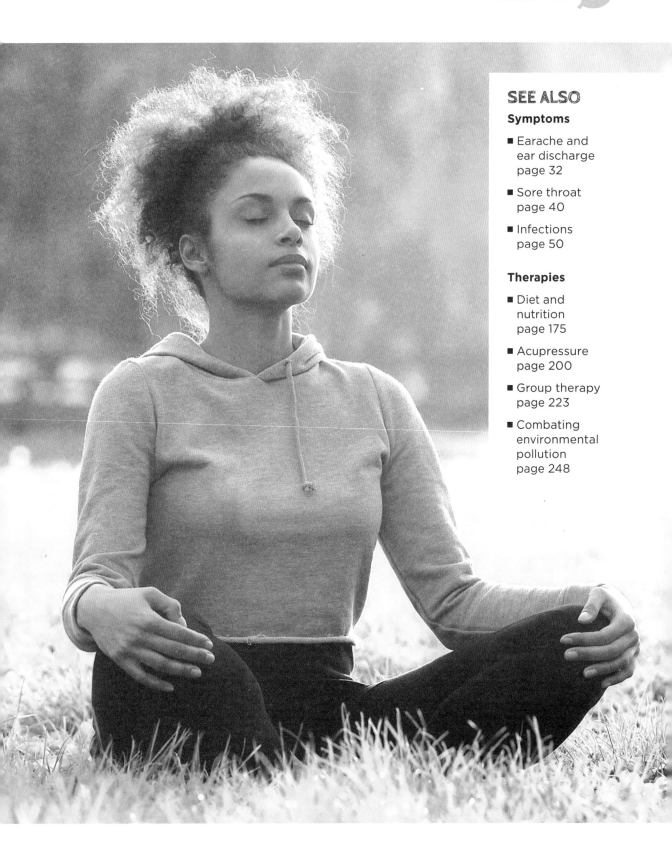

SEE ALSO

Symptoms

- Earache and ear discharge page 32

- Sore throat page 40

- Infections page 50

Therapies

- Diet and nutrition page 175

- Acupressure page 200

- Group therapy page 223

- Combating environmental pollution page 248

DIZZINESS

There is often confusion about the symptoms of dizziness, vertigo, tinnitus (ringing in the ears), and loss of balance. Dizziness may come primarily from some effect on the inner ear, the related part of the brain, or even the emotional system.

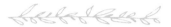

Conventional Therapies

- Blood pressure check

- Physical examination of the head and neck area

- Audiogram, if there is any suspicion of hearing loss

Although the symptoms may be similar, it is important to distinguish between them in order to locate and treat the cause.

Dizziness: This can mean several things—giddiness, faintness, wooziness, and even elation! Dizziness can be related to high or low blood pressure (from any of several causes), and is also found in the context of emotional shock.

Vertigo: This refers to the specific sensation of whirling or spinning. If you close your eyes and have someone turn you around and around for 15 seconds, you will probably experience vertigo.

Tinnitus: This is a steady, usually high-pitched, musical tone that is perceived as coming from within one ear or the head generally. It is often known as ringing in the ears.

Loss of balance: This can result from slipping or putting a foot out carelessly, or it can occur without any apparent cause.

When vertigo, tinnitus, and loss of balance occur simultaneously, you may fall down or crash into a nearby wall! You probably have a temporary disturbance of the semicircular canals in the inner ear, an important organ in determining balance and spatial orientation.

COMPLEMENTARY THERAPIES
Stress management

Since these symptoms may be connected with circulatory dynamics, it is important to look at stress and lifestyle issues. Alterations in the circulation are often connected with excessive stress.

Diet and nutrition

Special things to look out for if you suffer regularly from dizziness are excess fat and salt in your diet and also excess body weight.

Acupressure

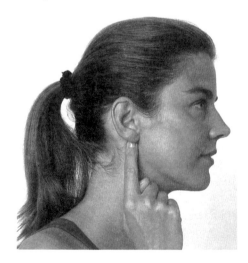

Stimulate the pressure point located behind the ear to give a stabilizing effect when feeling dizzy.

SEE ALSO

Symptoms

- Blood pressure page 59
- Loss of consciousness page 122
- Anxiety and panic page 130
- Diabetic symptoms page 158

Therapies

- Exercise page 180
- Massage page 186
- Breathing therapy page 190
- Meditation page 215

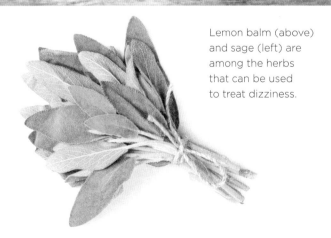

Herbal therapy

The following herbs are among those that have been found useful for dizziness.

- Balm
- Hawthorn
- Lavender
- Peppermint
- Rue
- Sage

Lemon balm (above) and sage (left) are among the herbs that can be used to treat dizziness.

MOUTH SYMPTOMS

The mouth is a very busy place where a number of things happen, such as chewing, smiling, speaking, breathing, salivation, and the beginning of digestion. It is therefore very important that the mouth be free of serious problems at all times.

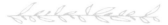

Conventional Therapies

- Periodic dental care
- Antibiotics and antifungal agents
- Local surgery

The first step to keeping your mouth healthy is to maintain a regular hygiene program, which should include regular visits to a dentist. However, a number of symptoms can arise in the mouth that require specific attention.

Chapped or cracked lips: Chapping is usually due to exposure to cold, wet weather and is best treated by your favorite lip balm. Cracking, particularly in the corners of the mouth, may signify vitamin and mineral deficiency, especially of the B-complex.

Sore spots or areas in the mouth: There are many kinds of "spots" in the mouth, from biting your cheek to cold sore (caused by a virus), most of which go away in a relatively short time. Thrush, a yeast infection caused by *Candida albicans*, appears as flat white patches in the mouth and other parts of the digestive tract. It is treated with antifungal drugs, but it is an important indicator of an imbalance in the population of normal bacteria in the body; it can occur after excessive use of antibiotics. A lump or spot in the mouth can be considered suspicious if it lasts more than a few days or grows bigger. Some dentists and their hygienists now give digital examinations of the mouth to detect these spots.

Toothache: Most toothache is due to infection at the root of a tooth. This is one situation in which an antibiotic can solve the problem. Root canal surgery may also be carried out, with variable results. Dental infections can be traced to a combination of improper diet (especially sugars, which corrode teeth) and inadequate self-care of the teeth.

Cavities (caries): Cavities in teeth are less of a problem now than in previous generations, but are still rampant in some sectors of society, notably at the lowest socioeconomic levels. Diet and self-care can do much to improve this area. Fluoride treatment is given a share of the credit by many for the overall reduction in caries in the population, but general improvement in diet is also cited.

Bad breath: There are many causes of bad breath (halitosis), including infection in the mouth and throat and sour stomach. People can have a bad taste in the mouth without its producing bad breath; the cause may be psychological or metabolic. The breath can clearly reflect a number of metabolic processes occurring in the body—conditions in the lungs, liver, kidneys, and bloodstream may be represented by breath odors.

"Having a regular dental check is the best way to prevent tooth decay. This applies to both children and adults."

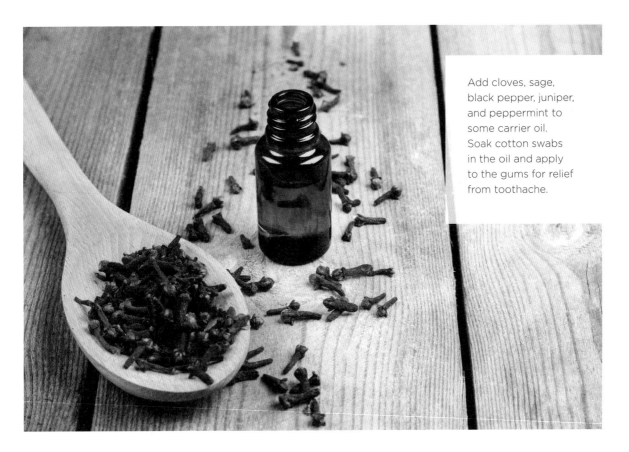

Add cloves, sage, black pepper, juniper, and peppermint to some carrier oil. Soak cotton swabs in the oil and apply to the gums for relief from toothache.

COMPLEMENTARY THERAPIES
Herbal therapy
- Balm (toothache)
- Caraway (halitosis)
- Clove (toothache)
- Dandelion (indigestion, bronchitis, and liver)
- Dill (halitosis and indigestion)
- Echinacea (halitosis, gum symptoms, and inflammation)
- Fennel (sinus and bronchitis)
- Garlic (sinus and bronchitis)
- Goldenseal (halitosis, gum symptoms, indigestion, inflammation, sore throat, and sinus)
- Peppermint (indigestion and liver)

Diet and nutrition
A properly balanced, nutritious diet supplemented appropriately by vitamins and minerals will go a long way toward preventing, as well as treating, many of the diverse conditions that contribute to unpleasant breath odors. A healthy, well-nourished person has clean, sweet breath. In general, complex foods—such as most meats—engage more metabolic processes for digestion, giving rise to certain odors. This is somewhat less true of fruits and vegetables, which are easier to digest.

Acupressure
Apply pressure to large intestine 4 for temporary relief from toothache.

Aromatherapy
- Sage, chamomile, fennel, and myrrh (to strengthen gums)
- Sage, black pepper, juniper, peppermint, and clove (toothache)

SEE ALSO
Symptoms
- Sore throat page 40
- Swollen glands page 42
- Infections page 50
- Cough page 66
- Indigestion page 152

Therapies
- Homeopathy page 244
- Naturopathy page 245

SORE THROAT

Sore throat is usually an indication of infection, which may be viral or bacterial. The soreness is often preceded by a sensation people describe as "scratchy." At this early stage, progression of the symptoms may be headed off if action is taken.

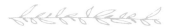

Conventional Therapies

- Antibiotics (inappropriate unless bacterial infection can be proven)
- Pain-relievers
- Rest

A gentle massage with sandalwood and other aromatherapy oils will help to soothe a sore throat.

These throat symptoms may herald the onset of a common cold or a much less common bacterial pharyngitis. Throat discomfort also occurs as a result of swollen glands in the front of the neck. Any number of external agents can also produce irritation of the throat when inhaled, including smoke, smog, dust, and chemicals.

At the onset of a sore throat, it is best to take plenty of rest, keep warm, and drink generous amounts of fluid.

COMPLEMENTARY THERAPIES
Diet and nutrition

In addition to the usual healthy diet program, one or two supplements have been found helpful early in the course of a sore throat, preferably in the "scratchy" stage. A lozenge containing 30mg of vitamin C and 15mg of zinc has been produced by at least one manufacturer, and has been found by many people to abort the development of a full-blown sore throat. The addition of extra vitamin C at this stage—up to 3,000 or 4,000mg per day for two to three days—seems to have a similar effect.

Herbal therapy
- Echinacea
- Goldenseal
- Marigold
- Red sage

Hydrotherapy
The use of steam will bring relief, either alone or with the addition of tincture of benzoin.

Acupressure
Press CV 22 or lung 10 to help soothe a sore throat.

Aromatherapy
- Gargle with two drops each of tea tree and sandalwood oil in water.
- Mix nine drops each of sandalwood and clary sage oils with seven drops of ginger and massage them into the throat, face, and upper chest.

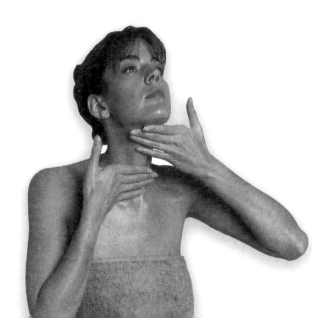

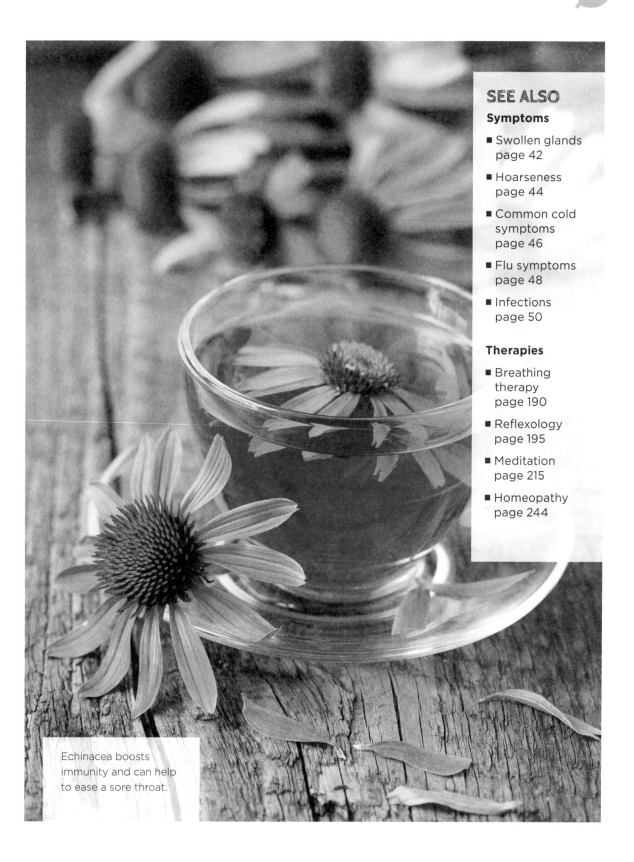

Echinacea boosts immunity and can help to ease a sore throat.

SEE ALSO

Symptoms

- Swollen glands
  page 42

- Hoarseness
  page 44

- Common cold
  symptoms
  page 46

- Flu symptoms
  page 48

- Infections
  page 50

Therapies

- Breathing
  therapy
  page 190

- Reflexology
  page 195

- Meditation
  page 215

- Homeopathy
  page 244

SWOLLEN GLANDS

Lymph glands or nodes are distributed around the body and act as part of its defense system against infection. Thus, they are an important part of the immune system, which also includes the liver, spleen, and bone marrow. When working to combat an infection, the lymph glands may become swollen.

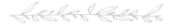

Conventional Therapies

- Antibiotics, fluids, and rest for infections (viruses do not respond to antibiotics)

- Various complex treatments for lymphomas and leukemias

The glands we notice most are those in the front of the neck, on either side of the windpipe, which become sore or swollen when the throat is infected. Other lymph glands are affected by other parts of the body; for example, those in the armpit or elbow may swell due to an infected cut on the hand. Bacteria travel up the arm through the lymphatics, tiny channels that connect the lymph glands, to be intercepted at these points. A "battle" ensues between the bacteria and the white blood cells, and this activity causes the glands to swell.

This can be described as regional defense. When glands are swollen all over the body, a generalized process involves all the glands. Virus infections, such as infectious mononucleosis ("mono"), act this way, as do blood disorders like lymphoma and some leukemias, but these are much less common in occurrence.

COMPLEMENTARY THERAPIES
Diet and nutrition
Vitamin C doses of 1,000–3,000mg a day are helpful in the prevention of colds and other infections.

Homeopathy
- Focusing ingredient: Echinacea purpurea 2x
- Accompanying ingredient: Belladonna 4x

Acupressure
The pressure point lung 11 is located on the outside of the thumb, $\frac{1}{16}$in (2mm) to the side from the base of the nail. Press hard and inward with a sharp pointed object, such as a toothpick, for 7–10 seconds.

LYMPHATIC SYSTEM
The main lymph glands that work to intercept infection in various parts of the body.

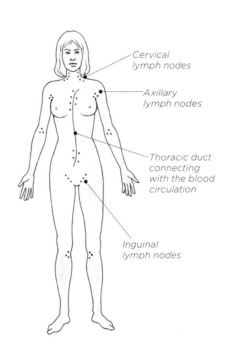

Cervical lymph nodes

Axillary lymph nodes

Thoracic duct connecting with the blood circulation

Inguinal lymph nodes

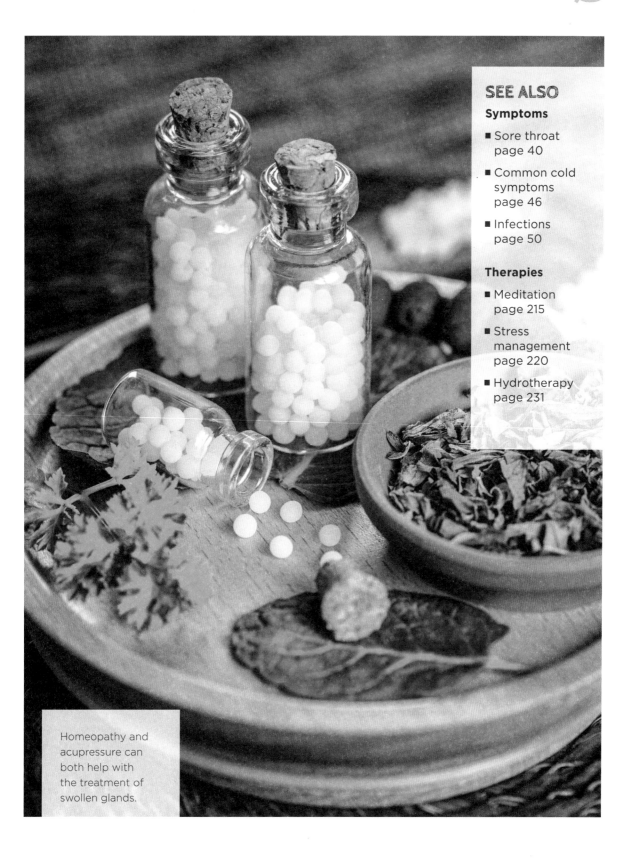

SEE ALSO

Symptoms

- Sore throat
  page 40

- Common cold
  symptoms
  page 46

- Infections
  page 50

Therapies

- Meditation
  page 215

- Stress
  management
  page 220

- Hydrotherapy
  page 231

Homeopathy and acupressure can both help with the treatment of swollen glands.

HOARSENESS

Hoarseness may be caused by anything that interferes with the normal operation of the vocal cords in the larynx, or voice box. Any infection or other inflammation of the voice box is called laryngitis.

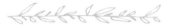

Conventional Therapies

- Treatment of any associated infection
- Voice rest
- Surgery

SEE ALSO

Symptoms

- Sore throat page 40
- Common cold symptoms page 46
- Flu symptoms page 48
- Infections page 50

Therapies

- Homeopathy page 244
- Combating environmental pollution page 248

Finding a definite cause is affected by the circumstances in which the hoarseness occurs, such as a common cold, and whether it is acute or chronic.

Infections: The most common infection to affect the larynx is the common cold. Others are bacterial infections of the throat and bronchial tubes, which may be primary, or complications of the common cold or the flu syndrome.

Growths: The most common growth to affect the larynx is called a polyp. This is a benign tumor that develops slowly until it reaches a size that is modest, but large enough to produce hoarseness. A small percentage of polyps undergo malignant change.

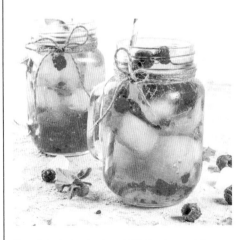

Raspberries are an excellent source of vitamin C and their leaves can be used to make a gargle to alleviate hoarseness.

Inflammation: A great many other things beside infections may lead to inflammation of the larynx. Probably the most common is overuse, which afflicts public speakers, singers, and the like, and can lead to polyp formation. Other causes are the inhalation of a variety of irritating substances in the air.

COMPLEMENTARY THERAPIES

Hydrotherapy

Inhaling steam is beneficial for inflammation related to hoarseness.

Diet and nutrition

In addition to the usual healthy diet program, supplementing with vitamin C to a level of 2,000–3,000mg per day may be helpful in combating inflammation.

Herbal therapy

The following herbs are useful for hoarseness, usually as a gargle. To prepare a gargle, steep the leaves of the plant as you would when making tea. Gargle with the liquid for around 10 seconds once every 3–4 hours.

- Coltsfoot
- Garden raspberry
- Goldenseal
- Mullein
- Plantain
- Slippery elm

"Hoarseness can be eased by inhaling steam, with or without the addition of herbs or essential oils. Control the steam with a towel over your head."

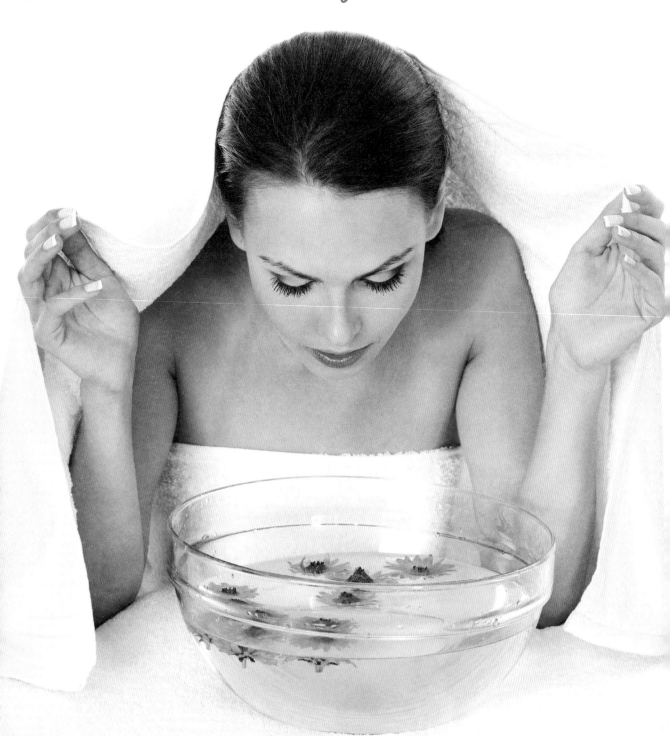

COMMON COLD SYMPTOMS

Symptoms of the common cold need little or no explanation to the average reader. They include sneezing, red, watery eyes, scratchy throat, cough, swollen glands in the neck, stuffy, runny nose, thirst, and mild fever.

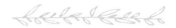

Conventional Therapies

- Rest, fluids, and pain-relievers
- Antibiotics (not appropriate unless there is a complication)

The common cold is caused by the rhinovirus and is known as a droplet infection, since the virus is usually passed from person to person via droplets in the air or droplets passed from hand to hand and hand to mouth. As the common cold is a viral infection, the use of antibiotics is not helpful, because antibiotics are only effective against bacteria.

A cold may be complicated by a secondary bacterial infection such as sinusitis, for which antibiotics may be effective. However, many people have found that by avoiding antibiotics altogether in this situation, they suffer fewer subsequent colds. This may be because the immune system becomes stronger without the use of antibiotics, or weaker because of their use.

COMPLEMENTARY THERAPIES
Aromatherapy

- Place one drop of eucalyptus oil on a tissue and inhale regularly to alleviate stuffiness. Try putting a drop on your pillow at night.
- Inhale steam to find general relief from cold symptoms. Use four drops of tea tree oil, four drops of eucalyptus oil, and two drops of peppermint and inhale the steam four times a day.
- Gargle one drop of tea tree oil in water to ward off colds.

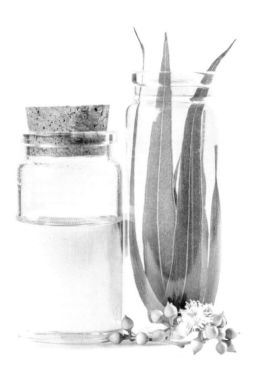

Sprinkling a drop of eucalyptus oil on a tissue and inhaling it helps to unblock a stuffy nose.

Reflexology

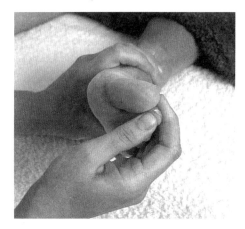

Cold symptoms can be helped by pressing each sinus point on the tips of the eight minor toes. Some sinus reflexes may be more tender than others. With sensitive pressure, the localized tenderness in the toe melts away, and you may feel immediate clearing of head congestion.

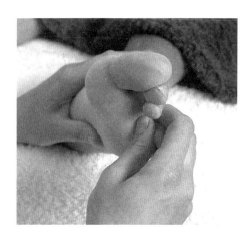

When the nose is congested, the eustachean tube from the middle ear to the back of the throat may be blocked. Gentle pinching of the corresponding reflex, between the third and fourth toes, can help to clear it. Support the foot with the other hand while you do this.

Diet and nutrition

High doses of vitamin C—3,000-4,000mg per day—for a few days at the very start of cold symptoms have been found to be extremely effective in heading off a cold or reducing the duration and severity of the symptoms. The usual healthy dietary program should prove helpful in avoiding colds altogether.

Acupressure

- Large intestine 4 and 20 are particularly useful for providing relief for a stuffy, runny nose.
- Lung 1 and 5 for "productive" cough and wheezing.
- Lung 10 and CV 22 for throat soreness.

Homeopathy

- Aconite 6x (sneezing)
- Euphrasis 6x (watery eyes)
- Natrum mur. 6x (runny nose)

Herbal therapy

- Boneset
- Elderflower
- Nepeta
- Peppermint
- Yarrow

A hot tea of equal parts of elderflower (below), peppermint, and yarrow is beneficial drunk at least three times a day. Add boneset if there is a fever.

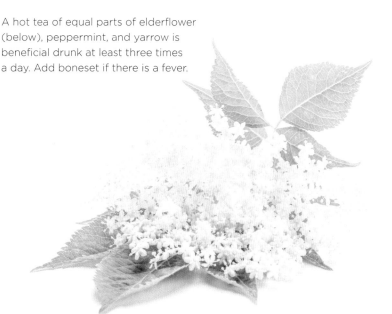

SEE ALSO

Symptoms

- Sinus headache page 27
- Eye symptoms page 28
- Earache and ear discharge page 32
- Sore throat page 40
- Swollen glands page 42
- Flu symptoms page 48
- Infections page 50
- Cough page 66

Therapies

- Therapeutic touch page 212
- Hydrotherapy page 231

FLU SYMPTOMS

"Flu" is a label that has been affixed to certain sets of symptoms in the past few decades, although it has been around for much longer. Earlier generations have had other labels for it, such as "the grip" or "la grippe."

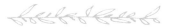

Conventional Therapies

- Light diet with appropriate fluid replacement
- Antispasmodic drugs
- Drugs to lessen pain and fever
- Bed rest

Flu is one of the less well understood clinical syndromes, partly because it is largely defined by each individual who experiences it, and partly because there is another condition called "influenza" that differs quite markedly from it.

Influenza: This is a serious viral illness that occurs in cycles of several years, so that a different strain prevails each year worldwide. Elderly and other susceptible people receive "flu shots" against this illness each year.

Flu: This is believed to be a viral illness with some of the same symptoms as influenza, but it lasts only one to three days, as a rule. The symptoms may be quite severe, but because the illness is so brief, serious complications rarely occur. Flu is a neighborhood illness, influenza a worldwide one. Flu symptoms fall into two general patterns; a person has either one type or the other: respiratory or gastrointestinal.

People with the respiratory type experience all the symptoms of the common cold, plus headache, muscular aches, and fever with shaking chills. People with gastrointestinal flu experience nausea, vomiting, abdominal cramping, and diarrhea, along with headache, muscular aching, and fever. It is virtually synonymous with viral gastroenteritis. It may be confused with food poisoning, but the latter generally lacks the aching muscles and fever.

COMPLEMENTARY THERAPIES
Aromatherapy

- Add four drops each of cedarwood and chamomile and two drops of ginger to water. Inhale the mixture in steam to treat a dry cough.
- Drink a glass of honey water with four drops of peppermint added for nausea.
- Add two drops each of geranium, juniper berry, and peppermint oils to a warm bath for diarrhea.

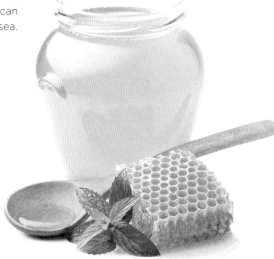

Honey water with peppermint can counter nausea.

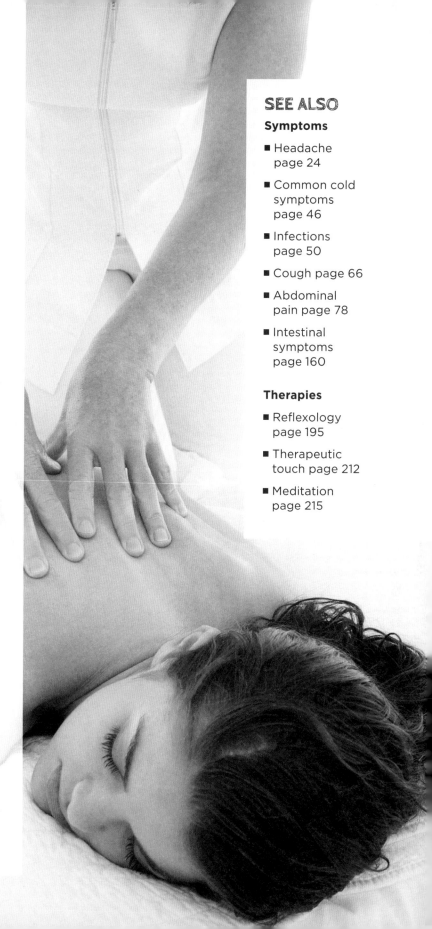

Herbal therapy

- Boneset, calendula, echinacea, garden violet, meadowsweet, sandalwood, and willow (fever)
- Marshmallow, coltsfoot, mullein, thyme, and wild cherry (cough)
- Belladonna, chamomile, peppermint, calendula, lavender, and fennel (cramps)
- Balm, calendula, peppermint, goldenseal, savory, and spearmint (nausea)
- Calendula, carrot, peppermint, garlic, coltsfoot, and meadowsweet (diarrhea)

Homeopathy

- Baptisia (gastrointestinal symptoms and extreme weakness)
- Eupatorium perf. ("aching bones")
- Gelsemium (heavy head, sore eyes, and fever with shaking chills)

Acupressure

Applying pressure to lung 7 and large intestine 4 when symptoms first appear will help to repel the infection. Press large intestine 11 to relieve fever and diarrhea and CV 12 to regulate digestion. Press stomach 25 for intestinal problems and diarrhea and stomach 86 to help diarrhea and digestion and to improve resistance to disease.

Massage

A massage with eucalayptus oil can be used to treat cold symptoms and aching limbs, and sandalwood will help remoisturize the dry skin that often accompanies colds and flu. Massage is also beneficial in the immediate aftermath of flu, when the person may feel "low" and irritable. In this case, use jasmine oil as an antidepressant or chamomile for relaxation.

SEE ALSO

Symptoms

- Headache page 24
- Common cold symptoms page 46
- Infections page 50
- Cough page 66
- Abdominal pain page 78
- Intestinal symptoms page 160

Therapies

- Reflexology page 195
- Therapeutic touch page 212
- Meditation page 215

INFECTIONS

The general subject of infection is intimately related to the discussion of immunity. One of the major tasks of the immune system is the detection, interception, and elimination of infectious agents. Anything that damages the integrity of that system increases the person's susceptibility to infection.

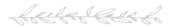

Conventional Therapies

- Antibiotic drugs
- Intravenous fluids
- Drugs to combat pain and fever
- Surgical drainage

If you are able to grow your own produce, avoid using chemical fertilizers and sprays.

There are a great many agents capable of producing such damage—in the air we breathe, the water we drink, and the food and other things we put in our mouths.

It is ironic that one of those agents is antibiotic drugs; while designed to eradicate infection, they also work in several ways to encourage it.

The use of antibiotics leads to drug-resistant strains of bacteria emerging as a result of adaptive mutation. This has led the drug industry to try to keep up by developing new antibiotics; some say this battle is being lost. Antibiotics upset the intestinal population of bacteria essential to our existence by killing off certain strains. Among the outcomes of this are deficiencies of certain vitamins and other nutrients because the relevant bacteria are not present to promote their digestion and absorption. Another effect is the overgrowth of yeasts and fungi, such as *Candida albicans*, which then attack tissues and organs.

People also tend not to take antibiotics for as long as they have been prescribed. This can and does lead to the killing off of the weakest organisms, while the strongest ones attack tissues with even greater force.

So there are strong arguments for avoiding antibiotics in all but serious situations. Many people find that the less they use antibiotics, the fewer situations arise in which they might be prescribed. The message here is that when we do not use them, our immune mechanisms probably act more efficiently to handle even large numbers of bacteria, preventing their colonizing in tissues.

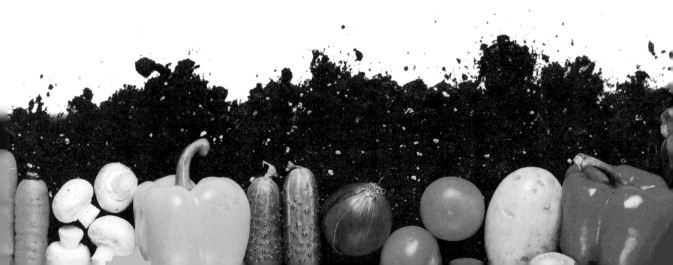

COMPLEMENTARY THERAPIES

Diet and nutrition

An optimal nutrition program is a key element in any strategy aimed at preventing and/or managing infections. Here are a few specific observations.

- Vitamin C has been shown in many studies to have preventive value in the common cold and other infections. A level of 1,000–3,000mg per day is not excessive. After the onset of an infection, a level of 4,000–6,000mg per day will combat the depletion of vitamin C that occurs with the combination of infection and stress.
- Sore throat symptoms are markedly relieved by the early use of zinc lozenges, 23mg, taken several times a day. Lozenges that supply a combination of zinc and vitamin C are widely available.
- Severe infections deplete stores of magnesium; therefore, supplementation is desirable.

Herbal therapy

- Berberine, a constituent of goldenseal, Oregon grape, and bayberry, is effective in a wide range of infections and has both antibacterial and antiviral effects in AIDS.
- Bromelain enhances tissue levels of antibiotics, if their use is required.
- Echinacea is known to be helpful in many infections.
- Garlic has antibiotic effects in AIDS.

Stress management

Infections often occur in the setting of emotional stress, so if you are prone to them, it would be well for you to think about your sources of stress, particularly in relationships at home and at work. If you do contract an infection, that is an additional stress to deal with, so it is best to start studying your stress situation when you are not aggravated by illness.

Meditation

Infections disturb many of the body's balances. The ability to connect with the calm center of being through meditation is very helpful in restoring lost balance. Find which method suits you best; this may be traditional yogic meditation or simply resting in a quiet room. It is preferable to find a method when you are well and then to practice regularly. If you do become ill, the path to that center will be clear and familiar to you.

Combating environmental pollution

If you are a gardener, avoid the use of chemical fertilizers and discourage their use by others. As a consumer, encourage alternative methods by buying produce certified as organic, or produced without chemical feed or fertilizers. Those containing antibiotics increase the incidence of drug-resistant bacteria that abound and increase the genetic pool of such bacteria. This means greater risk of infection for all.

Therapeutic touch

Massage can calm tension and ease pain when infection disrupts well-being, but sensitive, caring touch and stroking can be especially valuable therapy in conditions such as AIDS, adding to feelings of strength and self-esteem.

SEE ALSO

Symptoms

- Symptoms relating to immune function page 166

Therapies

- Imagery page 218
- Bach flower remedies page 236
- Homeopathy page 244

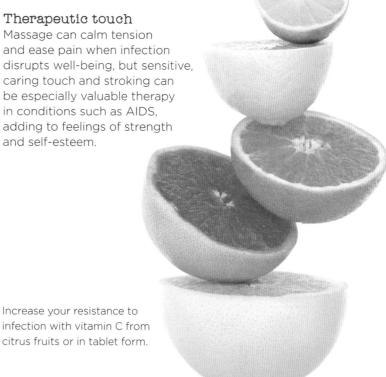

Increase your resistance to infection with vitamin C from citrus fruits or in tablet form.

FATIGUE

Fatigue is a generalized feeling of tiredness, in contrast to feeling sleepy (desiring sleep) or feeling weak or faint. It is overall weariness, and extreme fatigue borders on exhaustion. It occurs in association with a wide variety of other symptoms, and its origin can be obscure.

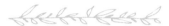

Conventional Therapies

- Based on history, physical examination, and laboratory testing

SEE ALSO

Symptoms

- Since fatigue can be associated with virtually any other symptom, you may wish to consult any other entry in the Symptoms section.

Fatigue did not receive a lot of attention as a symptom until recent years, when a condition that was ultimately labeled Chronic Fatigue Syndrome (CFS) started attracting notice. The typical CFS person is a young intelligent female (or occasionally a male) who has previously been very active and energetic, but who now experiences a dramatic loss of energy, a need to lie down often, and intolerance of social activities. Episodes of low-grade fever occur at intervals. The incapacity that results is quite severe, requiring long periods of rest and abstinence from gainful work. The duration of the illness can be from weeks to years. CFS has been studied a lot, but there is still no single theory as to its cause.

Other conditions with which fatigue is usually associated include wasting diseases, such as advanced cancer and AIDS; metabolic conditions, such as diabetes and thyroid disorders; and emotional states, such as marked anxiety and depression. Therefore, fatigue is an unspecific symptom that reflects a loss of vital energy. It is treated conventionally in the context in which it occurs.

COMPLEMENTARY THERAPIES
Stress management

The presence of severe fatigue and an illness that it may represent are additional stresses to those already present in everyday life. Thus it is very important to sort out such things as personal quarrels or disputes, or at least to put them on "hold," to allow the body to get on with the business of healing.

Meditation

There is a need for energy conservation after a bout of severe fatigue so that the body can restore the many balances that have been disturbed. The ability to connect with the quiet, calm center of our being is invaluable in this situation.

Acupressure

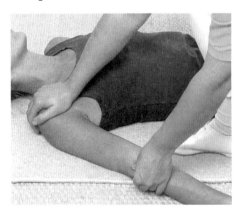

Increase stamina by working large intestine 10, found at three fingers' width below the elbow crease, on the line running up from the forefinger. This discourages fatigue and promotes feelings of well-being.

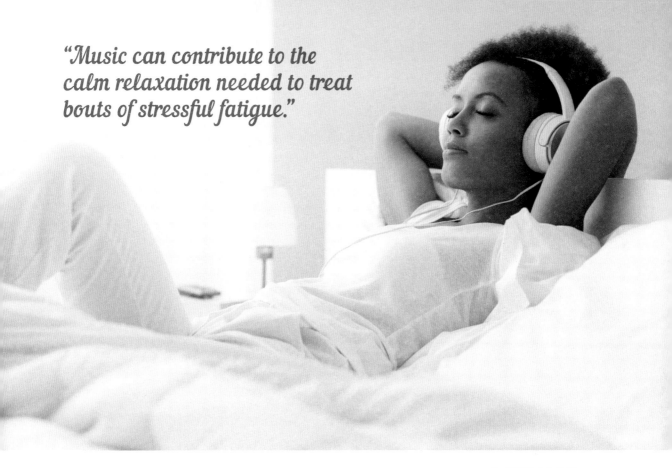

"Music can contribute to the calm relaxation needed to treat bouts of stressful fatigue."

Music therapy

Listening quietly to music at home relieves tension, and in music therapy groups sound is used to help people relax and share their problems.

Diet and nutrition

Underlying virtually all instances of excessive fatigue is a deficiency of one or more essential nutrients. Every effort should be made to supply missing nutrients. In those conditions with diminished appetite, a strong argument can be made for vitamin and mineral supplements, since there will be multiple deficiencies, especially given the added stress of the accompanying illness.

- Vitamin B1 deficiency has been found to be present in a high proportion of people with severe fatigue. In Chronic Fatigue Syndrome, 250mg per day for a month has resulted in marked improvement of symptoms.

- In CFS, there is a lowering of magnesium in red blood cells. Supplementation has produced 50–80 percent improvement.
- In CFS, the use of fish oils results in improvement in a high percentage of cases.
- Fatigue has been traced to high sugar intake, which decreases vitamins and other nutrients.
- The fatigue of premenstrual syndrome is much improved by vitamin B6.
- Fatigue has been noted to improve in people who have mercury amalgam fillings removed.

Exercise

It has been said that "fatigue is exercise deficiency," meaning that physical exercise leading to conditioning tends to diminish feelings of fatigue. In virtually all cases, nutritional changes would also need to be made before improvement occurs.

SEE ALSO

Therapies

- Massage
  page 186

- Reflexology
  page 195

- Imagery
  page 218

- Art and color
  therapy
  page 225

- Hydrotherapy
  page 231

- Aromatherapy
  page 232

- Herbal therapy
  page 240

- Homeopathy
  page 244

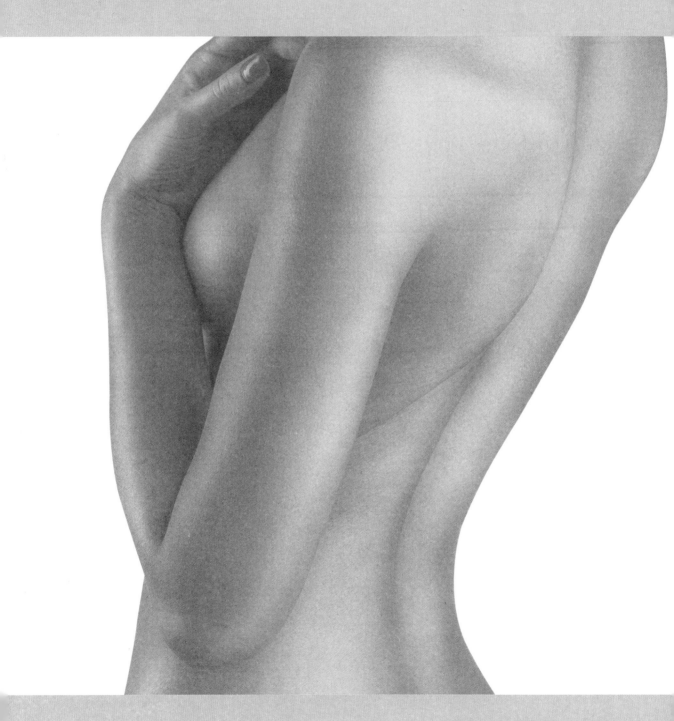

CHEST & BACK

CHEST PAIN

There is probably no area of the body where a tentative home diagnosis is more important than in chest symptoms, chiefly because of the possibility of heart attack. It is not necessary to make a sophisticated diagnosis at home, but rather to decide whether the symptom is serious or not.

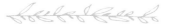

Conventional Therapies

- Improving the circulation of blood in and around the heart

- Improving oxygen exchange in the lungs

- Managing pain itself

Several kinds of pain and discomfort are experienced in the front of the chest. The person at home who is trying to decide what to do about a particular pain needs to answer a few straightforward questions, similar to those that would be asked in any emergency room.

Pain in the front of the chest is most likely to be serious if:
- It covers a relatively large area.
- It is tight or squeezing rather than sharp.
- It is associated with nausea, sweating, or faintness.
- It is accompanied by tingling pain in the arm, neck, or jaw.

If all or most of these criteria are present, the prudent course is to arrange transport to the nearest emergency facility for further diagnosis, observation, and treatment. If in any doubt at all, always see a doctor.

If the chest discomfort is not of this type, it may be quite safe to remain at home and deal with the symptom there. If the pain is sharp and quite localized, it is probably something relatively superficial. Look for a skin rash, which might signify the onset of shingles. The pain may be caused by a muscular strain, or, if there has been an accident, a cracked rib. There may be a clear association with digestive activities, or the very familiar feel of heartburn or indigestion. There are also several syndromes involving ribs, rib cartilages, and the intercostal nerves that run around the chest and can produce this kind of pain.

The most notable recent advances in the management of chest pain have come in the field of cardiology, where research clinicians like Dr. Dean Ornish have demonstrated over suitably long trial periods that the actual obstructions in the coronary arteries diminish under intensive treatment programs. Such programs are designed to be followed at home without supervision, and must be followed indefinitely if satisfactory results are to be obtained.

The programs feature diets specifically designed for cardiovascular disease and provide techniques for achieving inner calmness. A level of physical activity tailored to each individual is also incorporated in the program.

"Chest pain during physical exertion may not be life-threatening, but needs immediate attention. See a doctor about any pain of unknown cause."

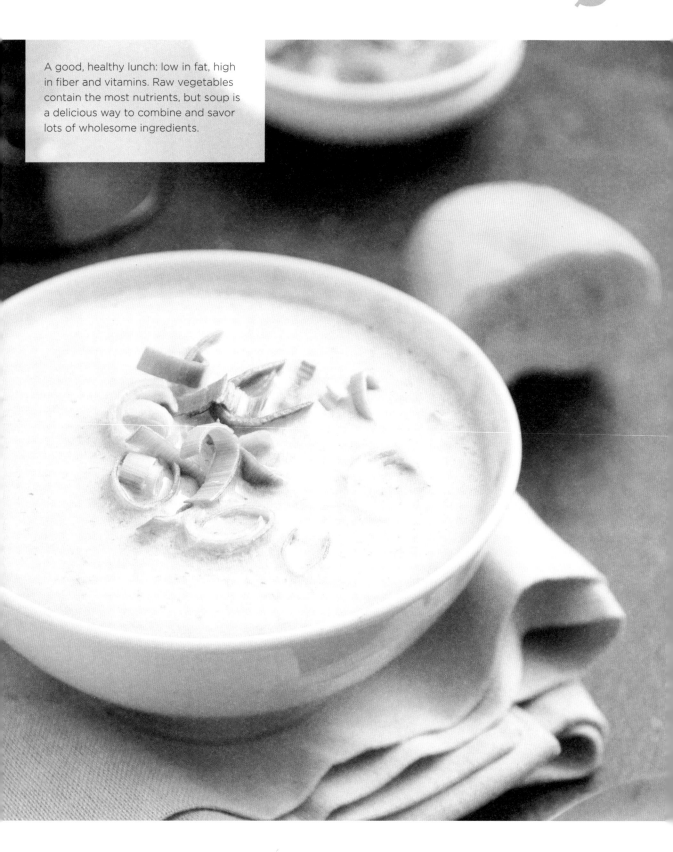

A good, healthy lunch: low in fat, high in fiber and vitamins. Raw vegetables contain the most nutrients, but soup is a delicious way to combine and savor lots of wholesome ingredients.

COMPLEMENTARY THERAPIES

Diet and nutrition

A diet program specifically for cardiovascular disease is one that prevents, or even reverses, the process of laying down fatty deposits in the lining tissue of arteries like the coronaries.

Such a diet will be very low in fat and high in fiber, as well as generous in raw fruits, vegetables, and whole-grain breads. It should also include supplementation of vitamins, minerals, and other substances that have antioxidant properties; these include vitamin C, vitamin E, beta-carotene, selenium, coenzyme Q, and zinc.

Meditation

Techniques for achieving inner calmness are many and varied. You can simply set aside time for your favorite relaxing activities, such as reading or painting. However, a deeper kind of meditation can reach the serenity that lies at your core, and it is this connection that can have a significant effect on your body's physiological processes. This can work with diet and exercise to arrest, and in some cases reverse, the course of degenerative changes in the body that are linked to coronary disease.

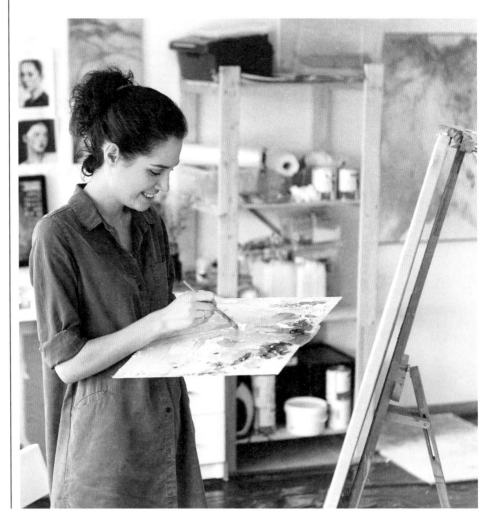

Enjoying a relaxing activity, such as painting, helps pain management and disease control.

BLOOD PRESSURE

Blood pressure means the pressure within the arteries (not the veins), which carry the blood pumped by the heart to all the tisues of the body. The pressure is uniform throughout the system of arteries.

Each time the heart beats, there is a spike of pressure; the reading at the top of this spike is called the systolic pressure. It is normally 120mm and tends to rise gradually as the arteries age and become less elastic, but this is not in itself considered serious. The pressure in the arteries between beats, when the heart is resting, is called the diastolic pressure and is normally 80mm. Any significant rise in this pressure can cause problems over time because it is the resting pressure in the system, and therefore the lowest of which the system is capable.

The immediate cause of this kind of pressure change, which we constantly hear referred to as hypertension or high blood pressure, is contraction of the tiny muscles in the walls of the smallest arteries, or arterioles, all over the body, thus narrowing their caliber and raising the pressure in the system. This happens whenever there is an increase in certain chemicals circulating in the bloodstream that are responsible for the tone of those tiny muscles. The brain and nervous system control the flow of these chemicals and we can control that flow voluntarily. Thus to a very significant extent we can control our blood pressure and reduce or eliminate hypertension.

Why should we care about our blood pressure? The main reason is that prolonged hypertension causes excessive wear and tear on the arteries, on which all our tissues depend for the delivery of life-sustaining blood. This wear and tear mainly takes the form of deposits called plaques or atheromas in the lining of the arteries. These plaques build up over time to the point where they can partially or completely obstruct the flow of blood to the tissue supplied by the artery. This situation is responsible for the vast majority of heart attacks, strokes, and kidney failure, and contributes to the complications of diabetes. So it is of the utmost importance that we know something about it and what we can do to prevent it.

For something as significant as hypertension, the early symptoms can be quite unimpressive. Initially, when blood pressure is wavering between normal and slightly elevated, there are no recognizable symptoms. Some people continue to have no symptoms until the artery-blocking process has begun. Others report nonspecific symptoms such as headache or dizziness. So there is no reliable way of telling whether blood pressure is high except to measure it.

Conventional Therapies

- Anti-hypertensive drugs, all of which have side-effects
- Low-salt and low-calorie diets
- Surgery

"Home-testing kits are now widely available for measuring blood pressure, which could provide a vital early warning of preventable disease."

SEE ALSO

Several options exist. You can have your blood pressure tested at intervals, either as part of a health checkup or at a special health screening center or event. Alternatively, you can learn to test it yourself. This has a built-in advantage, in that some people get falsely high readings when they are tested by someone else. Blood pressure begins to be a little high when the resting diastolic pressure is over 85mm, and above that, the higher the reading, the greater the cause for concern. The normal range of pressure is between 125/85 and 90/60, with readings just beyond that range being of questionable significance. (The systolic pressure is the higher number and is usually given over the diastolic pressure.) Low blood pressure is rarely as serious as high blood pressure and is often temporary. Some people consistently have readings in the lower part of that range. This is normal, especially if everything else is healthy.

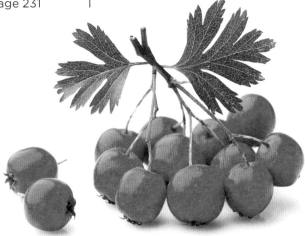

Hawthorn berries help to improve circulation, regulate heartbeat, and lower blood pressure.

COMPLEMENTARY THERAPIES
Stress management

Chronic difficulties in relationships at home and in the workplace comprise the major stresses that people encounter in our culture. In addition, we are subject to internal stresses arising from childhood events and other occurrences. Hundreds of studies have confirmed the correlation between stress and high blood pressure. Trying to manage the stress in your life can bring great benefits.

Diet and nutrition

An optimal nutrition program is essential for the maintenance of overall balance that results in normally controlled blood pressure. Here are a few particulars.

- Being overweight is responsible for 20–30 percent of the incidence of hypertension.
- Drinking more than three units of alcohol a day correlates with high blood pressure. (One unit equals a single measure of spirits, a medium-sized glass of wine, or one pint of beer.)
- Stopping smoking substantially reduces the risk of stroke (a metabolic effect).
- Increasing the intake of calcium, magnesium, potassium, and vitamin C reduces blood pressure.
- High dietary sodium (e.g. eating a lot of salty foods) correlates with high blood pressure.

Meditation

Numerous studies lasting many years have confirmed that meditation techniques practiced regularly have a consistent effect in lowering blood pressure. The evidence here is very strong. All you need to do is to find what method suits you best, then carry it out daily. The results are obtained by achieving calmness and inner balance.

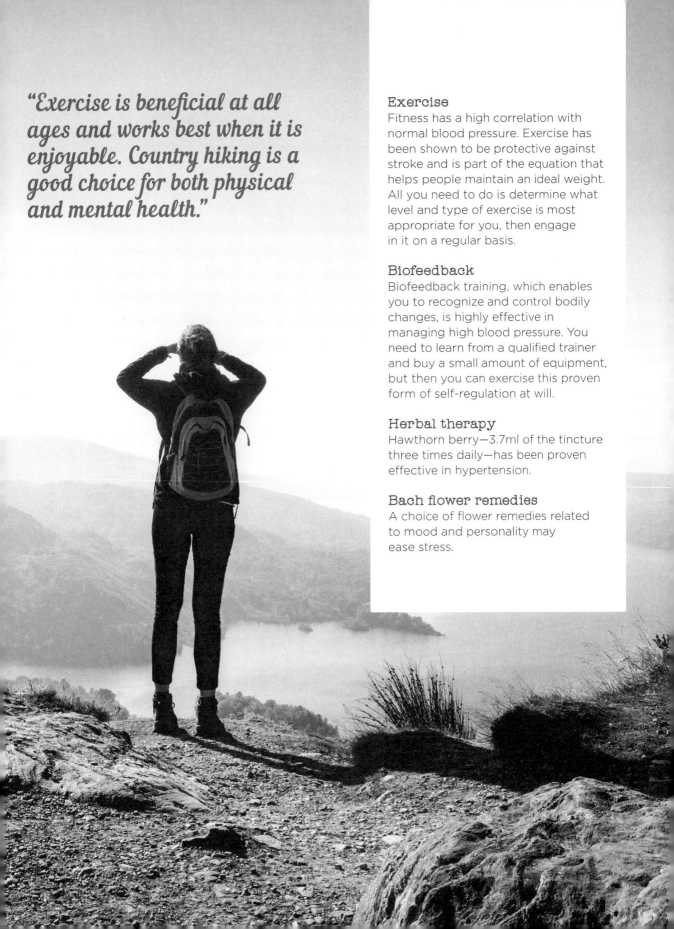

"Exercise is beneficial at all ages and works best when it is enjoyable. Country hiking is a good choice for both physical and mental health."

Exercise

Fitness has a high correlation with normal blood pressure. Exercise has been shown to be protective against stroke and is part of the equation that helps people maintain an ideal weight. All you need to do is determine what level and type of exercise is most appropriate for you, then engage in it on a regular basis.

Biofeedback

Biofeedback training, which enables you to recognize and control bodily changes, is highly effective in managing high blood pressure. You need to learn from a qualified trainer and buy a small amount of equipment, but then you can exercise this proven form of self-regulation at will.

Herbal therapy

Hawthorn berry—3.7ml of the tincture three times daily—has been proven effective in hypertension.

Bach flower remedies

A choice of flower remedies related to mood and personality may ease stress.

CHOLESTEROL LEVELS

The subject of cholesterol is quite high on the list of health-related items discussed currently, but there is a great deal of misinformation on the subject. A high cholesterol level is technically a sign, not a symptom, but it merits discussion here simply because it is so widely discussed, and often misunderstood.

Conventional Therapies

- Low-fat, low-cholesterol diets
- Drugs, most of which have harmful side-effects

The significance of various cholesterol levels in people's blood has been the subject of much debate and thousands of studies in medical and scientific circles over the past 40 years, and new facts are being turned up all the time. These facts do not always enlighten the discussion, but merely broaden the range of possibilities. The question always needing to be answered is whether, or to what extent, the blood level of cholesterol is related to the incidence of blood vessel diseases and to the disability and death that may result from them. The question is more complicated than it seems at first, and clear answers are hard to come by.

Here are a few important facts about cholesterol that are generally ignored in public discussion.

- 80 percent of the cholesterol in our tissues is manufactured in the body (from fat, protein, and certain forms of carbohydrate) and only 20 percent enters the body ready-made in food.
- Increased blood cholesterol usually results from increased synthesis within the body, not from modest increases in dietary cholesterol.
- Cholesterol is an essential substance in the body, not a demon as it is often portrayed. It is a vital constituent of the walls of every cell

in the body, and is the precursor of the adrenal steroid hormones, which regulate everything, from bone and glucose metabolism to inflammation and immune responses.

It is clear from the above that Nature intended us to have a generous supply of cholesterol. It is only when we have excessive amounts that the body has trouble off-loading it. So it is important that we do not have an antagonistic attitude toward it—cholesterol is us!

Another concept that we need in order to understand the cholesterol question is that there are several kinds of cholesterol, depending on how it is hooked up with certain fats and proteins. This is complicated, so to put it in the simplest way, we only need to know about HDL and LDL cholesterol, which together make up most of our cholesterol count.

HDL cholesterol (HDL for high-density lipoprotein) makes up about one-third of the total count. It has a protective effect against the formation of the plaques that can invade blood vessels and block the flow of blood. A helpful thing to watch is the ratio of total cholesterol to HDL cholesterol. The national average risk of coronary disease correlates with about a 5:1 ratio, so you want to be better than that. For example, if your total cholesterol is 200 and your HDL

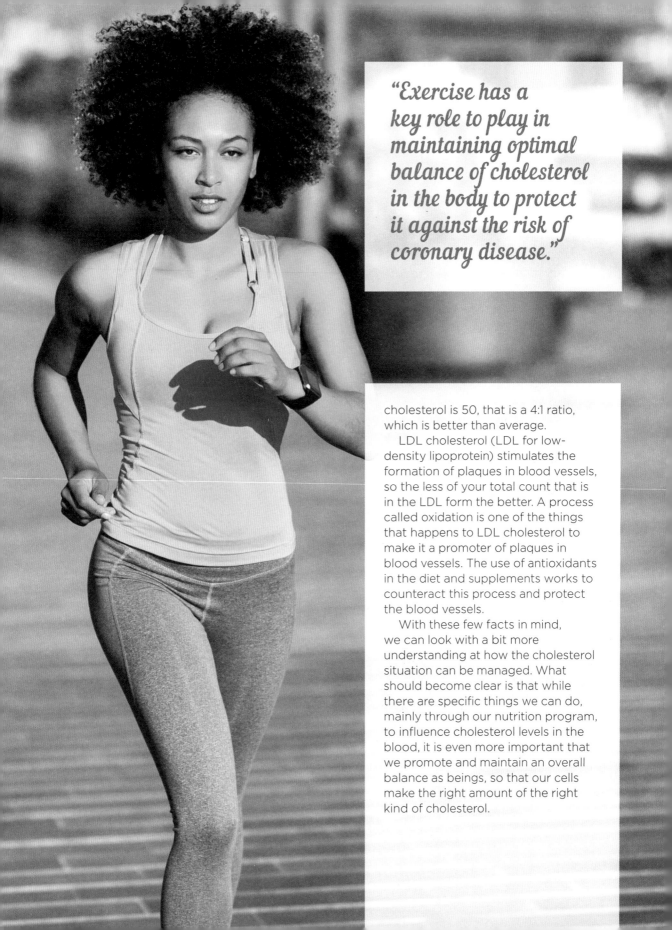

> "Exercise has a key role to play in maintaining optimal balance of cholesterol in the body to protect it against the risk of coronary disease."

cholesterol is 50, that is a 4:1 ratio, which is better than average.

LDL cholesterol (LDL for low-density lipoprotein) stimulates the formation of plaques in blood vessels, so the less of your total count that is in the LDL form the better. A process called oxidation is one of the things that happens to LDL cholesterol to make it a promoter of plaques in blood vessels. The use of antioxidants in the diet and supplements works to counteract this process and protect the blood vessels.

With these few facts in mind, we can look with a bit more understanding at how the cholesterol situation can be managed. What should become clear is that while there are specific things we can do, mainly through our nutrition program, to influence cholesterol levels in the blood, it is even more important that we promote and maintain an overall balance as beings, so that our cells make the right amount of the right kind of cholesterol.

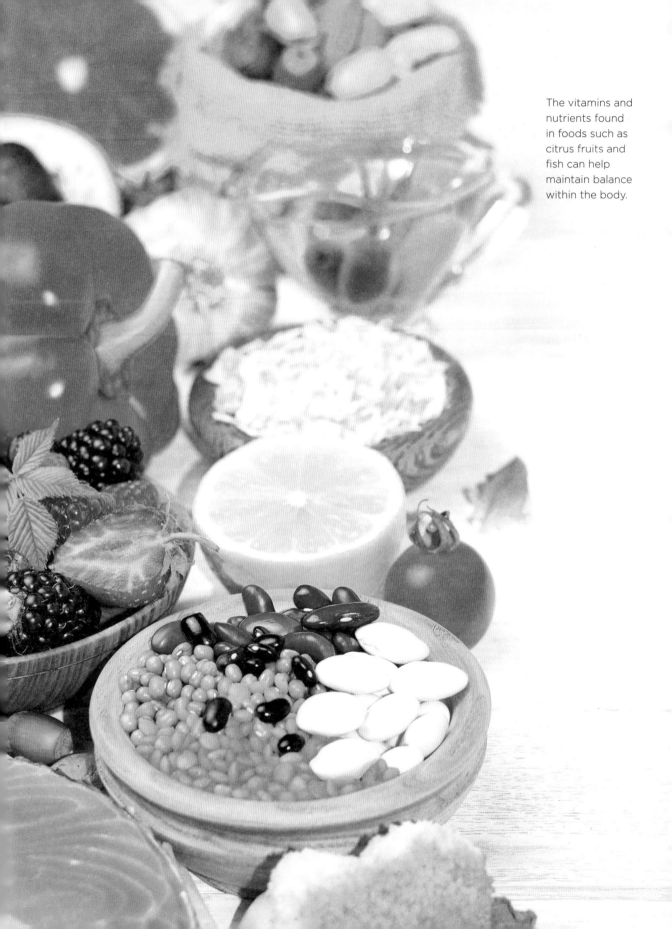

The vitamins and nutrients found in foods such as citrus fruits and fish can help maintain balance within the body.

COMPLEMENTARY THERAPIES

Exercise

Exercise is part of the equation that helps keep the body in balance. Specifically, exercise has been shown to lower LDL cholesterol and raise HDL cholesterol.

Diet and nutrition

An optimal nutrition program is of the utmost importance in maintaining a balance that promotes optimal levels of total cholesterol and other substances in the body. Here are some specific observations on the subject.

- Magnesium lowers total cholesterol and LDL-C and raises HDL-C.
- Niacin (500—1,000mg per day) lowers total cholesterol and LDL-C and raises HDL-C.
- Vitamin C in doses as low as 500mg per day raises HDL-C and lowers total cholesterol.
- Eggs (up to seven per week) have been found to have no significant effect on total cholesterol and can be safely eaten by healthy people.
- Vitamin B6 lowers LDL-C.
- Copper raises HDL-C and lowers LDL-C.
- Fish oils raise HDL-C.
- L-carnitine lowers total cholesterol and LDL-C and raises HDL-C.

Herbal therapy

- Amla (Indian gooseberry) lowers total cholesterol and LDL-C.
- Garlic (600–900mg per day) lowers total cholesterol.
- Gum guggula lowers total cholesterol and LDL-C and raises HDL-C (a lot!).
- Sesamin from sesame seeds lowers total cholesterol.

Stress management

The state of arousal provoked by stress hinders the body's task of maintaining healthy cholesterol levels. It is therefore beneficial to practice relaxation and anger management techniques.

Meditation

Transcendental meditation has been found to lower cholesterol when practiced regularly over a period of several months.

SEE ALSO

Symptoms

- Chest pain page 56
- Blood pressure page 59
- Eating disorders page 142
- Weight disorders page 146

Therapies

- Reflexology page 195
- Yoga page 204
- Imagery page 218

It is important to notice when you become stressed and to learn how to manage this.

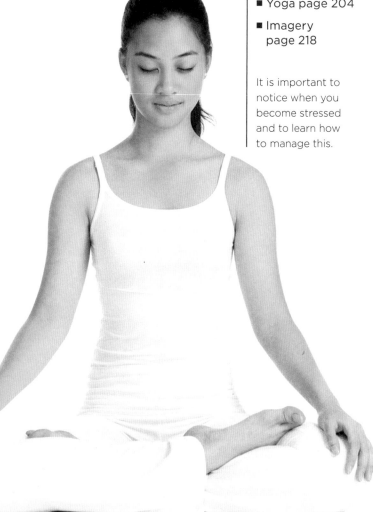

COUGH

Coughing is stimulated by anything that activates the cough reflex. This is made up of nerve receptors that are located along the respiratory tract well down the bronchial tube at the back of the throat, and of nerve channels leading to the brain and back to the glottis and respiratory muscles. The glottis closes during a cough and the respiratory muscles contract to force air past the closed glottis.

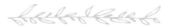

Conventional Therapies

- Antibiotics for infection
- Drugs

The nerve receptors are "tickled" by various stimulators, and the cough "scratches the itch." The purpose of the reflex is to expel instantly anything that might cause obstruction of the airway. However, it also responds to many things that do not have the potential to obstruct, but simply the quality of producing local irritation.

- Inhaled irritants such as noxious gases, smoke, chemicals, and even water (e.g. when swimming) can trigger coughing.
- Food, liquid, or even saliva inhaled during eating is a common cause of coughing. This is what happens when you get something "down your Sunday throat." It can be serious if a chunk of food is inhaled, which is why the Heimlich maneuver can be life-saving.
- Secretions from the lining of the bronchial tree resulting from infection can be irritants. These lead to episodic or chronic coughing, depending on the nature of the infection.
- Bleeding into the respiratory tract can cause coughing. This may be due to an infection, but is also a warning signal that a tumor may be present.

Note that coughing is also a common symptom of asthma.

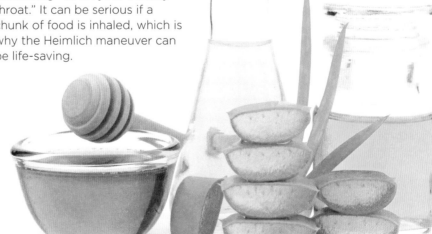

The combination of aloe vera and honey can help ease scratchy coughs.

COMPLEMENTARY THERAPIES

Herbal therapy

- Put two teaspoonfuls of dried hyssop in a cup of boiling water, steep for 10 minutes, then strain and drink.
- Put 25–30 drops of tincture of mullein in a small amount of boiling water and drink three times a day.
- Thyme, in the form of tea, helps to move out mucus.
- The juice of aloe vera mixed with an equal part of honey is particularly good for a scratchy cough.

Aromatherapy

The use of inhaled steam can liquefy mucus and reduce irritation.

- Place three drops of eucalyptus oil and three drops of hyssop oil in a basin of steaming water, and inhale the steam as long as it lasts, controlling the steam with a towel over your head.
- Place a few drops of tincture of benzoin in a steaming kettle or basin and inhale it.
- Another good blend is three drops each of cypress and juniper and a drop of ginger.

Diet and nutrition

- Vitamins A, C, and E are helpful in conditions that cause coughing.
- Zinc lozenges, also available with vitamin C, are beneficial.

Hydrotherapy

A bath or shower that creates lots of steam can ease coughing, and hot packs applied to the throat or chest are soothing. A humidifier or steaming kettle in the room can also help.

Combating environmental pollution

Atmospheric pollutants are an increasing source of irritation to the airways, and apart from avoidance, it is important to work for improvements in air quality.

Reflexology

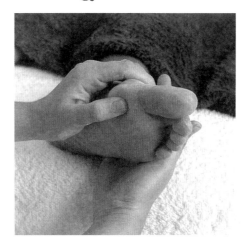

The throat and thyroid reflex is the padded area under the first (big) toe. "Walk" the thumb across it in varied directions at the first sign of a cough.

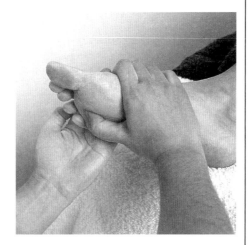

Ease back the toes to access the raised area that represents the chest reflex. Thumb-walk all over it to help release the congestion of a "chesty" cough.

SEE ALSO

Symptoms

- Hoarseness page 44
- Common cold symptoms page 46
- Flu symptoms page 48
- Infections page 50
- Chest pain page 56
- Symptoms relating to immune function page 166

Therapies

- Breathing therapy page 190
- Aromatherapy page 232
- Homeopathy page 244
- Combating environmental pollution page 248

WHEEZING AND SHORTNESS OF BREATH

Wheezing describes noisy breathing that has a high-pitched musical character; it tends to be more noticeable on the out-breath of the respiratory cycle. Constriction of the smaller bronchial tubes, the bronchioles, is the usual cause of wheezing.

Conventional Therapies

- Treatment of infection
- Drugs to relieve bronchospasm
- Supplemental oxygen

The bronchioles contain a muscular coat like that of a blood vessel, allowing them to dilate or constrict. When constriction is prolonged, it is called bronchospasm. This situation produces a sensation of breathlessness, or shortness of breath. This in turn leads to anxiety and panic, which escalates the shortness of breath, establishing a vicious circle. It is most characteristic of asthma, but it occurs in other situations where asthma is not a major factor. Allergenic substances in the air are a significant cause of bronchospasm.

Shortness of breath can also be produced by causes other than bronchospasm. These include chronic infection in the bronchial tree, leading to thickening of the bronchioles and ballooning of the tiny air sacs (emphysema); swelling of the lung tissues with water, as in congestive heart failure; and pressure exerted by tumor masses on the air passages.

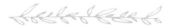

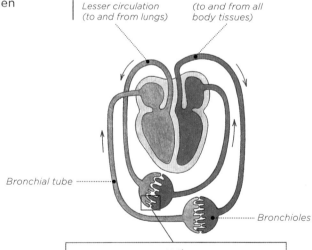

Lesser circulation (to and from lungs)

Greater circulation (to and from all body tissues)

Bronchial tube

Bronchioles

De-oxygenated blood from tissues via heart

Oxygenated blood in tissues via heart

Air

CO_2 out

CO_2 in

AIR SAC

OXYGENATION OF BLOOD IN THE LUNGS

Damage to the bronchial tubes affects the lungs' air sacs, reducing oxygen in the blood.

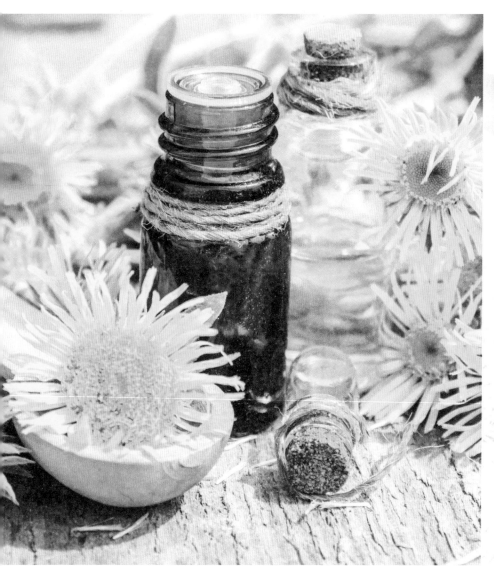

SEE ALSO
Symptoms
- Infections page 50
- Cough page 66
- Anxiety and panic page 130

Therapies
- Exercise page 180
- Alexander technique page 185
- Breathing therapy page 190
- Acupressure page 200
- Stress management page 220
- Combating environmental pollution page 248

COMPLEMENTARY THERAPIES
Aromatherapy
A few drops of the following oils, when inhaled from a tissue, may be effective. You can determine which blend is best for you and use the same blend in carrier oil for massage, especially on the chest and back.
- Eucalyptus
- Frankincense
- Lavender
- Sage

Herbal therapy
- Coltsfoot can be used for asthma, bronchitis, and emphysema.
- Elecampane is a very useful herb as it deals with asthma, bronchitis, and emphysema.
- Ephedra and thyme are of general benefit for these symptoms.
- Licorice is effective for bronchitis.

A tincture of elecampane flowers is a good natural therapy for wheezing and shortness of breath.

BREAST SYMPTOMS

Nowadays the breast, a source of joy when nourishing a child, can be the focus of concern, confronted as we are with a constant stream of information about breast cancer and its latest treatment. There are also a number of other issues, from the effects of the contraceptive pill to mammograms and premenstrual syndrome.

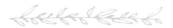

Conventional Therapies

- Combinations of hormone preparations
- Tranquilizers
- Surgery

Breast health is, of course, closely related to overall health, so the best way to prevent breast problems is to maintain a healthy lifestyle. This involves eating a healthy diet, exercising appropriately, maintaining inner calm, and dealing effectively with external stresses. This may sound like a big order, but as the benefits are great, it is not as difficult as it seems! With good health as the motivation, anyone can work on these areas on a daily basis.

The value of good nutrition to a woman's reproductive system cannot be overemphasized. It is especially important to avoid excessive fats, to eat lots of fiber, and to maintain a body weight that is within a healthy range. The appropriate use of vitamins and minerals as supplements helps by providing antioxidants and other important nutrients.

In some people, specific breast symptoms occur. Let us look at the most common ones.

Breast lumps: First of all, women should examine their breasts themselves. There are many local clinics where you can get instruction if you are not sure how to do it. If you examine regularly and there is a lump, you will be the first to discover it. A large percentage of breast lumps do not indicate cancer. Even so, this is your signal to seek medical opinion, and you will probably be advised to have a mammogram. You are placing yourself at certain risk if you do not follow medical advice about a mammogram or whatever subsequent treatment is advised. Do not be in too much of a hurry, though. It is perfectly safe to say you want to think about it for a few days to allow you to talk to a partner or friends and plan your next step in a calmer frame of mind. But do not delay it too long.

Swelling of the breasts: Your breasts may swell as part of the menstrual cycle, and you will know what is normal for you. If abnormal swelling occurs—and it is rare outside of pregnancy—always have it checked medically.

Discharge from the nipple: A little discharge can be normal with sexual stimulation. Anything beyond that, aside from lactation, should be checked, especially if there is discoloration.

Premenstrual syndrome (PMS): This is a complex of symptoms, including irritability, tension, depression, lethargy, incoordination, breast tenderness, headache, edema, bloating, and acne. In addition to general measures, regular aerobic exercise has been found to diminish symptoms significantly, as has supplementation with calcium, magnesium, and vitamin B6.

Examine your breasts once a month and have any abnormality checked out.

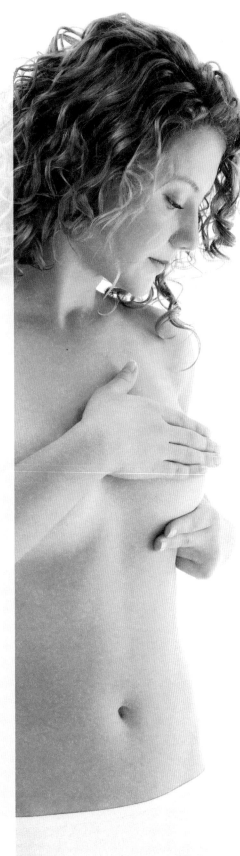

COMPLEMENTARY THERAPIES

Imagery

Imagery techniques that involve focusing on peaceful mental images to engender bodily calm can be especially helpful in diminishing the stress associated with the occurrence of breast cancer.

Exercise

Swimming is recommended for breast health, as are good posture and proper breathing.

Diet and nutrition

Diet is of particular importance where the health of the breast is concerned, since it so closely parallels the health of the person as a whole. Study carefully the section in Therapies dealing with diet (page 175).

Breast Cancer

- According to many authorities writing today, more than 50 percent of breast cancers can be shown to be diet-related.

- A 20 percent reduction in fat in the diet is effective in reducing breast cancer incidence.

- Increasing the intake of fiber to 25g per day is effective in reducing breast cancer incidence.

- Other factors shown to be effective in the prevention of breast cancer are reduction of stress, cessation of smoking, and avoidance of the use of estrogen and progesterone preparations.

SEE ALSO

Symptoms

- Fatigue page 52

- Menstrual symptoms page 86

- Sleep-related symptoms page 125

- Anxiety and panic page 130

- Depression page 134

Therapies

- Breathing therapy page 190

- Reflexology page 195

- Yoga page 204

- Therapeutic touch page 212

- Meditation page 215

- Stress management page 220

- Hydrotherapy page 231

BACK AND NECK PAIN

Pain in the back and neck is the most common cause of incapacity and disability in America and Britain. Many clinics deal with nothing but back pain, and a multitude of medical specialists have joined in the effort to deal with the problem, but it still goes on, causing as much pain and disability as before.

Conventional Therapies

- Pain-relieving medication
- Antispasmodic medication
- Advice about rest and work
- Physical therapy or surgery

Back pain arises from a number of different sources and for different reasons. Here we are talking mainly about the pain that arises from the muscles, ligaments, tendons, bones, and joints of the back itself. Keep in mind, however, that pain can be referred to the back from other areas and body systems. When pain in the back is steady and unrelated to movements, consider this possibility and look for other symptoms.

Pain arising from the structures in the back tends to be sharp, related to movement, and causes some limitation of mobility. Pain in the low back can radiate to one or both legs, sometimes with numbness or tingling in the lower leg or foot. This may be due to pressure on a nerve running from the back into the leg, which may be caused by a bulging invertebral disk or slippage of one vertebra on another. Similarly, a pain radiating into the arm may signify pressure on a nerve from the neck.

Inflammation and spasm of the muscles themselves is another cause of pain. This can be due to a strain or injury, or to chronic overuse of a muscle. Spasm or tightening of a muscle is usually due either to this kind of trauma or to the protective action of a muscle in preventing a part from moving.

COMPLEMENTARY THERAPIES
Exercise

Gentle moving and stretching, especially while in a warm bath, will help in maintaining muscle tone, if they can be done within the limits of significant pain. However, adequate rest for the painful area is also important. Find the position of least discomfort when resting, but remember that prolonged rest will decondition the muscles. This will cause problems by reducing muscle strength, thus opening the way for muscle strains and joint dislocations. This in turn will extend the period of recovery required to bring the muscles back to full strength.

Alexander technique

The Alexander technique helps to prevent or alleviate back pain by improving posture and breathing, releasing tension, and enabling you to use your body in a more natural, relaxed, and efficient way.

"The misery of back pain afflicts most people at some time, from many causes. Complementary therapies can help prevent and reduce pain."

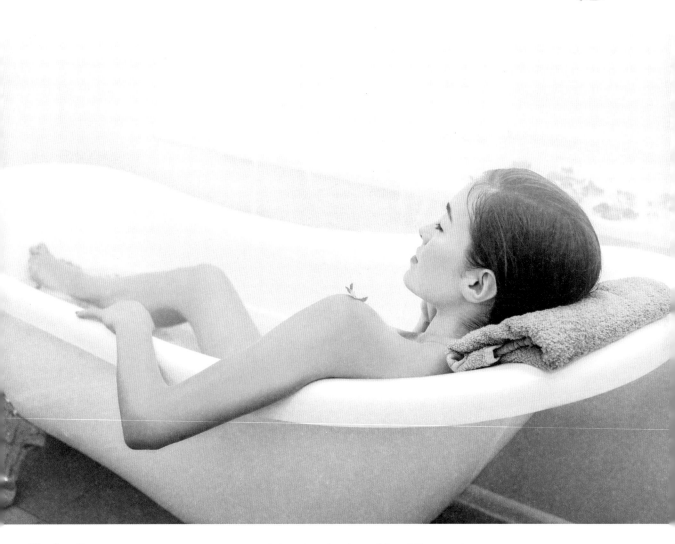

Hydrotherapy

Hot baths are a favorite in any and all situations, but especially helpful for back and neck pain. A hot bath promotes relaxation of the muscles and of the whole body. It also allows easier movement of the affected part than is possible in the air, since the water partly neutralizes gravity.

Aromatherapy oils, such as chamomile, juniper, lavender, or eucalyptus, can be added to the bathtub water to increase the relaxing effect. The oils can be used equally effectively in a compress applied to the painful area.

Hot and cold contrast bathing is best used after the first 48 hours of injury. It stimulates blood flow and thus brings the body's healing forces into the area. Apply a hot shower to the affected part for a minute, then splash cold water on it for 30 seconds. Repeat the process for five minutes. Cold packs are useful in the first 48 hours of a muscular injury. Apply to the affected area for periods of 20 minutes, with 20-minute rest periods in between. The packs help to combat swelling and spasm, and have the added benefit of numbing pain. Hot packs are good against localized stiffness—a covered hot-water bottle will do the trick. The packs can be used in conjunction with massage or passive stretching.

The soothing effect of a hot bath relieves the stress of pain and eases sore movement.

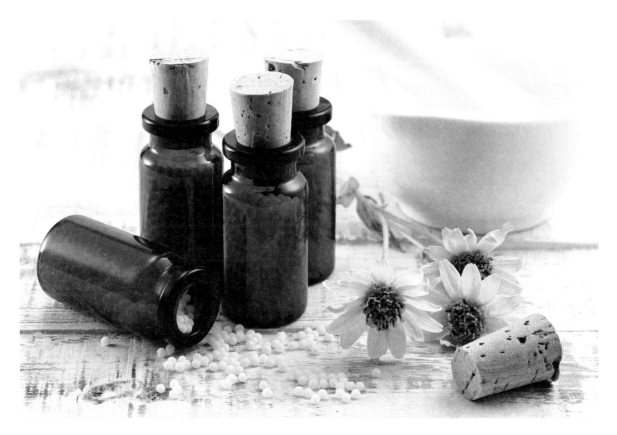

Arnica, in either tablet or topical cream form, is an effective homeopathic remedy for relieving back and neck pain.

Homeopathy

Arnica montana and St. John's wort (*Hypericum*) are two outstanding preparations used homeopathically. They are available both in tablet and in topical cream form, and can be used in combination with other products. Both give prompt and often lasting relief in quite severe muscular and ligamentous pain. As a cream, either can be applied locally, with a gentle, massaging motion.

Meditation

Find relaxation. The use of relaxation techniques is very helpful in combating the tendency to "tighten up" when pain strikes. After the acute phase is over and recovery is taking place, think how you can prevent pain from reccurring in the future. Considerations such as physical conditioning and weight control may come into the picture for you.

Stress management

Control of pain is of primary importance here, not only for comfort, but also because pain leads to muscle spasm, which in turn leads to more pain. In the acute stage of a painful injury, it may be necessary to use an over-the-counter pain-reliever. It is also very important that the person in pain has understanding friends or members of the family who can provide physical and emotional support.

Herbal therapy

- Guaiacum, Jamaican dogwood, St. John's wort (*Hypericum*), and valerian can give effective pain relief.
- Black willow, meadowsweet, devil's claw, white poplar, and wild yam are useful anti-inflammatory remedies.

Yoga

The various positions in hatha yoga are designed to bring about a balance among all the muscle groups of the body, within the context of mental, emotional, and spiritual serenity. This has proven beneficial for many who have suffered from chronic back pain.

Massage

Deep massage of the muscles of the neck and back serves several purposes. It reduces spasm of the muscle itself, which lessens pain, and also the traction applied by the contracted muscle at its attachment to other structures. The ultimate result is relief of pain, together with overall relaxation and a sense of well-being that in turn enhances the level of pain relief.

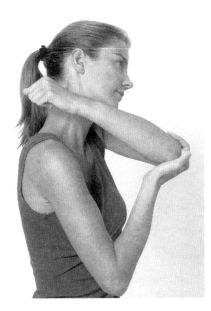

For relief from shoulder tension, support your working arm at the elbow and bang your shoulder, especially toward the neck, with the underside of your relaxed fist. This may sound fierce, but you can monitor the pressure. It is deeply calming.

Acupressure

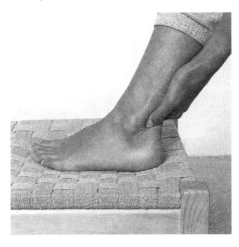

To strengthen the lower back, press kidney point 3 between the inner ankle and the Achilles tendon.

Reflexology

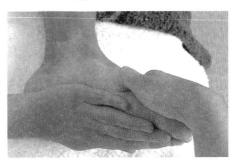

For upper back problems, thumb-walk along the cervical and thoracic spinal areas. These are located on the inside edge of the foot, starting under the first (big) toe and extending along the ball of the foot as far as the middle of the instep.

SEE ALSO

Symptoms

- Chronic pain page 19

- Joint pain page 94

Therapies

- Diet and nutrition page 175

- Breathing therapy page 190

- Tai chi page 208

- Therapeutic touch page 212

- Biofeedback page 228

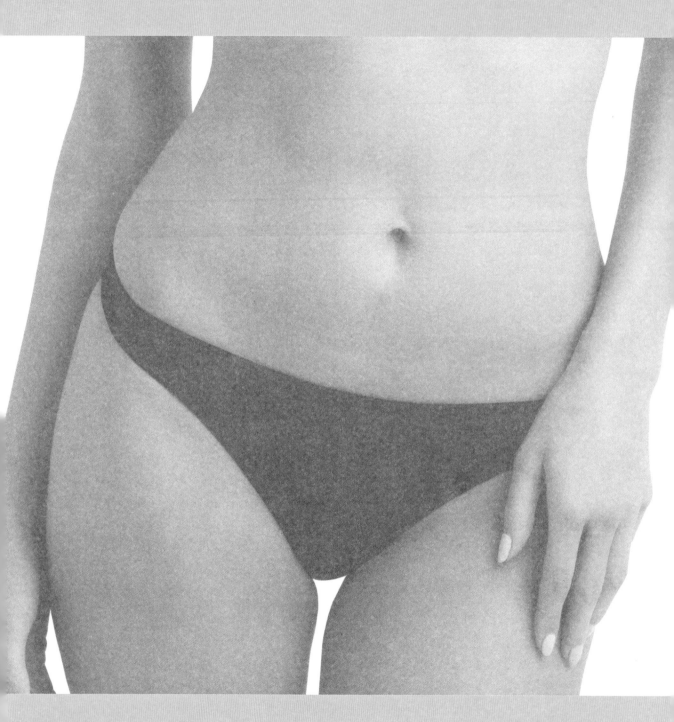

ABDOMEN & PELVIS

ABDOMINAL PAIN

Pain in the abdominal area can arise from the abdominal wall or from the structures lying within. In this area the sufferer often has a good sense of whether the pain's origin is superficial or deep. There are also a number of other clues, including location, digestion, and the type of pain and its relation to movement.

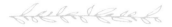

Conventional Therapies

- Antispasmodic drugs
- Pain-relieving drugs
- Surgery

Herbal teas, such as mint and cinnamon, can be soothing and relaxing, and bring relief from abdominal pain.

Pain arising superficially may be due to inflammation or compression of the superficial nerve trunks; this pain is likely to be sharp and localized. An example is shingles, caused by the herpes zoster virus, which may have an accompanying linear skin rash. (Shingles can occur in other parts of the body as well.) Pain coming from muscles and soft tissues has a sore, aching character and may be related to movement; a strained abdominal muscle is a common example.

Pain arising from within the abdominal cavity is produced by situations that cause direct pressure on, or stretching of, pain-sensitive structures. Internal masses, such as cysts and tumors, most often produce direct pressure. Stretching of tissue is generally due to intestinal spasm or obstruction of a passage, as happens with a kidney stone or a gallstone, with distension of an internal organ resulting. This may or may not cause the abdomen to appear swollen. If such a situation is suspected, medical opinion is essential.

When faced with abdominal pain at home, the first thing one wants to know is whether the problem is serious or not.

As a rule, one should seek medical help in the following situations.

- The pain is severe and shows no sign of letting up.
- There is a marked swelling or tenderness to touch associated with the incidence of pain.
- There is prolonged nausea and vomiting or any vomiting of blood.
- There is disturbance of consciousnes with prolonged reduction in the amount of fluid intake.
- There is prolonged diarrhea or any suggestion of dehydration.

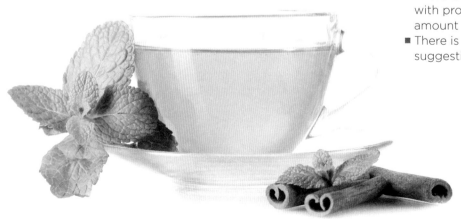

COMPLEMENTARY THERAPIES

Herbal therapy

Any combination of the following herbs may be prepared as a tea in the usual way. Simply find the combination that works best for your condition.

- Chamomile
- Cinnamon
- Fennel
- Ginger
- Lemon balm
- Peppermint

Meditation

Deep relaxation may be a valuable key to the relief of abdominal stress. Practice your chosen method every day when you are well so that you can turn to it with confidence when feeling distressed.

Hydrotherapy

Warm and hot baths are beneficial in cases of abdominal discomfort. Intestinal spasm is often relieved and overall relaxation achieved.

Stress management

Examine your lifestyle and try to regulate situations giving rise to stress and anxiety that contribute to pain and inhibit efforts to mitigate it.

Acupressure

CV 12 tones and regulates the digestive system. Stomach 36 tones the whole body via the digestive system and stomach 25 is helpful in treating intestinal problems, especially diarrhea.

Diet and nutrition

Avoid or reduce the intake of coffee and alcohol, which are gastric irritants. Eat regular, modest meals containing fresh ingredients and consume them in a calm atmosphere, where you can take time to relax and enjoy your food.

Reflexology

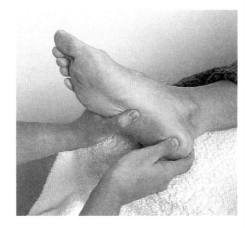

Abdominal pain resulting from emotional upset can be eased by supporting the middle of the foot with one hand and thumb-walking firmly over the bottom of the heel with the other.

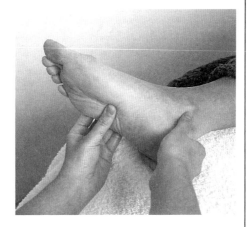

For constipation, thumb-walk clockwise up the ascending colon and across the transverse colon on the right foot, and then across and down on the left foot to push waste out of the body.

SEE ALSO

Symptoms

- Bloating page 80
- Anxiety and panic page 130
- Eating disorders page 142
- Indigestion page 152
- Intestinal symptoms page 160

Therapies

- Therapeutic touch page 212
- Homeopathy page 244

BLOATING

The abdomen is the only part of the torso that can be distended to accommodate changes in volume in the interior of the body. A small amount of distention may be part of the ebb and flow of internal events and not noted by the conscious mind. Beyond that point it may be recorded as a distress signal.

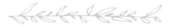

Conventional Therapies

- Antacid, antispasmodic, and anti-gas medication

- Gastric or rectal tube to release trapped gas

- Surgery

Herbal teas such as chamomile can help to settle the stomach and relieve bloating.

A bloated feeling in the abdomen can be caused by one or more of a variety of conditions.

Simple overeating: It is common to feel "stuffed" after eating heavy foods or a large meal.

Being overweight: When one's clothing is getting progressively tighter, there is often a sensation of chronic discomfort. Suspect excess weight if you no longer fit into last year's clothes!

Indigestion: This is common after the ingestion of spicy, greasy, or otherwise indigestible food; it is also seen when the body's production of digestive enzymes is lowered.

Accumulation of gas: Intestinal gas, a normal by-product of digestion, is sometimes present in excessive amounts or becomes trapped among loops of intestine.

Accumulation of fluid: This occurs in certain cases of heart or liver failure.

Inflammation: Any part of the intestinal tract can become inflamed as a result of irritation or neurochemical action in the body. Gall bladder disease is said to be associated with bloating.

Loss of peristaltic action: Known as paralytic ileus, this is when the muscular action of the intestinal wall slows or stops, usually as a result of illness or following abdominal surgery.

Obstruction: Blockage in any part of the bowel can produce bloating. The causes vary from constipation to adhesions of tissue after surgery and tumors.

Leakage from a blood vessel: This can result from injury to the abdomen or from blood vessel disease.

Leakage from a hollow organ: Examples include perforated ulcer and appendix, and ulcerative colitis.

COMPLEMENTARY THERAPIES
Diet and nutrition

Overeating, being overweight, indigestion, and accumulation of gas can be influenced by changes in your dietary patterns. In general, eating three modest meals per day, eating fresh rather than packaged foods, seasoning with herbs rather than a lot of salt and spices, and reducing the amount of fat in the diet will probably help you if you have any of these symptoms.

Some people have more trouble than others with certain foods. One possible reason is allergy or hypersensitivity to a food, which can be pinpointed by allergy testing or an elimination diet. Another possibility is that the body is producing less than optimal amounts of digestive enzymes, which sometimes happens as we get older. In this event, supplementing the diet with replacement enzymes may help.

Hydrotherapy

Warm baths often bring relief from simple gas conditions. Gentle enemas can bring relief if constipation is the major cause of the bloating. You can buy equipment for an enema at the drugstore and safely administer it yourself. Be gentle—use warm water or mild soapy solution and avoid stronger solutions. Note that this does not deal with the cause of constipation, but only stimulates bowel movement.

Acupressure

Applying pressure to CV 12 or 17, liver 3 or 13, stomach 36 or 44, or spleen 6 can help alleviate bloating.

Herbal therapy

- Cramp bark soothes spasms and relieves cramps.
- Chamomile is relaxing and acts as a gentle antispasmodic.
- Goldenseal is antispasmodic and a tonic to the mucus membrane lining the bowel.
- Peppermint is both antispasmodic and anti-inflammatory.

SEE ALSO

Symptoms

- Abdominal pain page 78
- Anxiety and panic page 130
- Indigestion page 152
- Jaundice page 156
- Intestinal symptoms page 160

Therapies

- Reflexology page 195
- Stress management page 220
- Homeopathy page 244

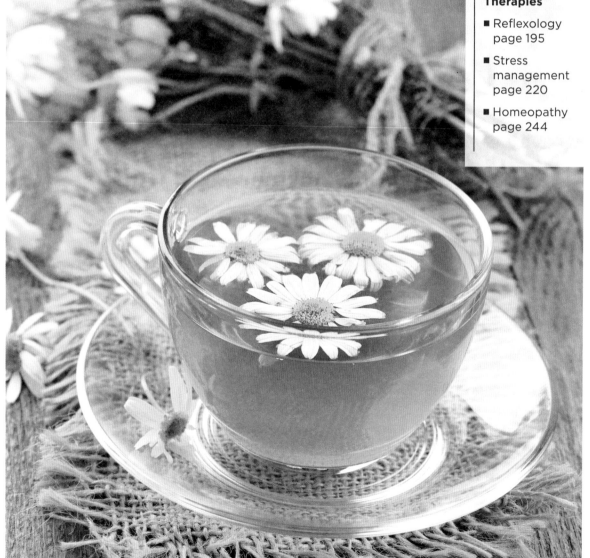

URINARY SYMPTOMS

The formation of urine by the kidneys is a vital process that most of us take for granted. The functional units of the kidneys are called nephrons. Each nephron contains a tiny blood vessel wound around an equally tiny kidney tubule, like two strands of wool in the same ball.

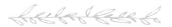

Conventional Therapies

- Antibiotics for infection

- Relief of obstruction with catheter (rubber tube) or surgery

- Removal of stone by dissolving, surgically, or other methods

- Surgical treatment of incontinence

- Surgical treatment of prostatic obstruction

- Combined treatment of prostate cancer

One little artery enters this ball, carrying blood laden with waste products and excess water, which pass into the tubule; another artery leaves it, carrying the cleansed blood, which returns refreshed to the general circulation.

The excess water and waste products from the blood form the urine, which drains away through a complex system of tubes to the bladder. This process is influenced by dozens of chemical reactions, enzymes, and biological processes.

The kidneys are the body's major regulators of fluid balance, acid-alkaline balance, nitrogen excretion, and concentration of dozens of minerals and other substances.

There are several major conditions that can prevent the kidneys from carrying out their functions. The little arteries in the kidneys can become blocked. Stones or tumors can block

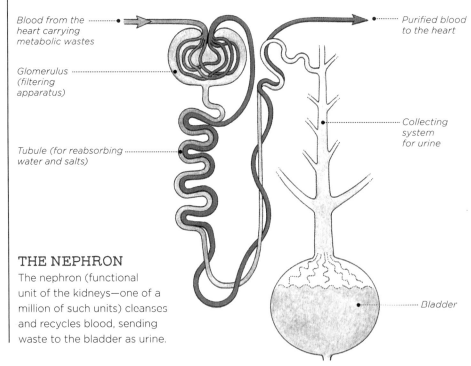

Blood from the heart carrying metabolic wastes

Glomerulus (filtering apparatus)

Tubule (for reabsorbing water and salts)

Purified blood to the heart

Collecting system for urine

Bladder

THE NEPHRON

The nephron (functional unit of the kidneys—one of a million of such units) cleanses and recycles blood, sending waste to the bladder as urine.

the urine ducts. In the male, swellings or tumor growths in the prostate gland, which is wrapped like a donut around the main urine tube as it leaves the bladder, can affect the function of the kidneys.

We tend to associate a certain group of symptoms with problems in the urinary tract, simply because they relate to the process of urination. In most instances, the correlation is reliable.

Urinary frequency and urgency: This is caused by irritability of the bladder due to irritation of its lining, or to overfilling following incomplete emptying.

Pain or burning on urination: These rather intense symptoms usually signify some degree of infection, or at least the presence of bacteria.

Discoloration or cloudiness of the urine: This can be caused by traces of blood, bacteria, crystals, and excessively concentrated urine.

Strong odor to the urine: This may be caused by stagnant urine due to incomplete emptying, concentrated urine, and foods such as asparagus.

Incontinence: This is not uncommon in women, especially during or after childbirth. The use of Kegel exercises (see Exercise, page 84) has been successful over many years in dealing with this problem without resorting to surgical approaches. Incontinence in men occurs mainly after prostate surgery and in advanced old age.

Obstruction of urine flow: This is usually due to prostatic enlargement or a stone in the urinary tract (usually painful), although congenital anomalies account for a small percentage of cases.

Water is the best daily provider of the plentiful liquid healthy kidneys need.

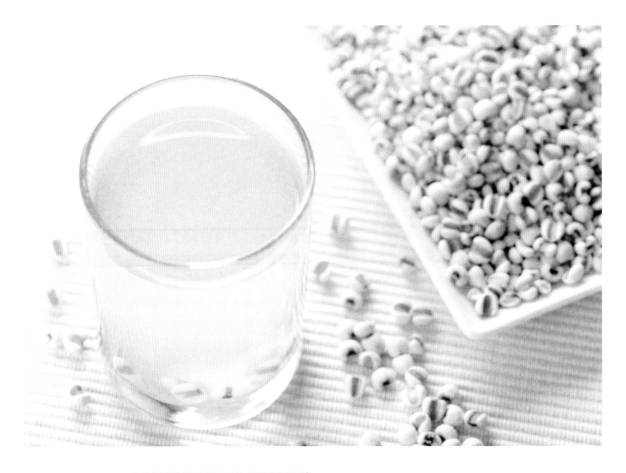

Drink barley water with honey and lemon to help cleanse the urinary system of infection and thus ease the pain of cystitis.

COMPLEMENTARY THERAPIES
Diet and nutrition
The health of the urinary tract depends on consistently following an optimal nutrition program. Make sure you have an adequate intake of liquids per day. In deciding this, a great many variables have to be taken into account, including the amount of sweat being produced by the body (which in turn depends on the ambient temperature and the amount of activity taking place) and the quantity of soups, stews, and other watery foods ingested. The best guides may be the thirst experienced and the amount and quality of urine passed. The quantity of liquid needed in the form of water and juices may be around four to eight glasses a day.

Take 200–400mg per day of cranberry concentrate in capsule form. This has been shown to interfere with the development of infection by setting up a barrier between the cells lining the bladder and bacterial cells trying to get a foothold. Taking the concentrate allows the ingestion of a large enough quantity to be effective; drinking cranberry juice does not. Avoiding coffee, tea, alcohol, spicy foods, and citrus fruits is also helpful for bladder infection (cystitis).

Exercise
Kegel exercises, named after the Californian surgeon who first used them, strengthen the pelvic muscles and are very effective in diminishing or abolishing stress incontinence. To find that group of muscles, the next time you are urinating, try to stop or slow down the flow of urine. This will indicate to you how strong those

muscles are. One way to do this exercise is to think of the pelvic muscles as a slow elevator, with the relaxed state as the first floor. Tighten the muscles slowly, as though going to the second floor. Then tighten a bit more (third floor). Count to five and move to the fourth floor. Then relax slightly, stopping in turn at the third, second, and first floors. Then go down to the basement, which means that the muscles even bulge outward a little, and then back to the first floor. This completes a "Kegel."

During active conditioning, do five Kegels 10 times a day, tapering off slowly as improvement occurs until you reach a level that maintains the improvement. Increase again whenever necessary.

Herbal therapy

- Sandalwood, echinacea, and goldenseal are effective for inflammation and infection.
- Saw palmetto (*Serenoa repens*) has been the subject of many studies in recent years that have established without doubt its efficacy in treating prostatic enlargement; it is used in doses of 160mg once or twice daily over four to six months. According to tests, three-quarters of those on this therapy have received significant benefit.
- Combine buchu, corn silk, couch grass, and marshmallow leaves, infuse, and drink a cupful every two hours to relieve cystitis.
- Simmer 4oz (115g) washed pot barley for 30 minutes in 1 pint (570ml) of water and strain. Add honey and cranberry or lemon juice. Drink half a cupful several times a day for cystitis.

Reflexology

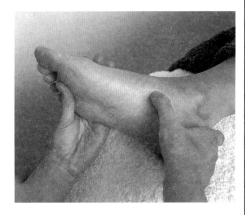

Thumb-walk with caution up the water tube and along the inside of the tendon, pulling back the first toe. Allow your thumb to press gently into the kidney point, just above waist level.

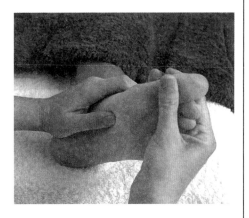

The cushioned pad halfway up the inside of the foot is the bladder reflex. When the bladder is empty, thumb-walk with care in lines, fanning up to the top of the foot and toward the toes.

SEE ALSO

Symptoms

- Infections page 50
- Diabetic symptoms page 158

Therapies

- Meditation page 215
- Stress management page 220
- Hydrotherapy page 231
- Homeopathy page 244

"All parts of the urinary system can develop infections, but though serious, they can usually be safely and effectively treated by natural means."

MENSTRUAL SYMPTOMS

The menstrual cycle becomes manifest at the onset of the menses (generally between the ages of 10 and 13). Under the influence of estrogen and progesterone, which are secreted in a cyclical fashion by the ovaries, menstruation—the shedding of the lining of the uterus—occurs at the end of a 28-day cycle, after which the uterine lining gradually builds up again throughout the following cycle.

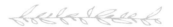

Conventional Therapies

- Hormone preparations to promote regular periods

- Surgery to promote ovulation

- Hormones for menopausal symptoms and prevention of coronary and bone disease

- Calcium and shell/bone preparations to counteract osteoporisis

Vitamin and other supplements can help you maintain a healthy menstrual cycle.

In mid-cycle one ovary discharges an ovum (ovulation), which travels down the corresponding fallopian tube into the cavity of the uterus. If the ovum is fertilized, it attaches to the lining of the uterus and pregnancy ensues. If it is not fertilized, the cycle proceeds until menstruation occurs.

These events are controlled by three hormones secreted by the anterior pituitary gland.

- Follicle-stimulating hormone (FSH) promotes the growth of the Graafian follicle, a cystic structure in the ovary that contains the developing ovum and secretes estrogen.

- Luteinizing hormone (LH) works throughout the cycle but is solely responsible for ovulation and the development of the corpus luteum from residual follicle cells. The corpus luteum secretes progesterone.

- Luteotropin or prolactin (LTH), along with LH, sustains the corpus luteum, either to the end of the cycle or throughout pregnancy.

The anterior pituitary gland, which produces these hormones, is in turn influenced by nerve impulses from the neighboring hypothalamus of the brain and by the cerebral cortex, the main switchboard of the brain, which processes input from all over the body as well as from the world outside. Thus the events governing female reproduction are under a wide variety of influences, both mental and physical, any of which can disrupt its smooth functioning.

Disturbances in the quality of these events may be reflected in any of the following symptoms.

Delayed start of menstrual periods: The age at which menstruation begins varies widely. If your child seems to be late starting, it is best to relax and wait, remembering that it is very rare for menses not to begin.

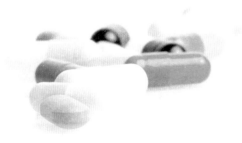

BRAIN

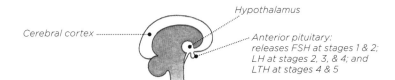

Cerebral cortex ....

Hypothalamus

Anterior pituitary:
releases FSH at stages 1 & 2;
LH at stages 2, 3, & 4; and
LTH at stages 4 & 5

OVARY

Stage 1: Maturation of follicle

Stage 2: Formation of estrogen in follicle

Stage 3: Ovulation and formation of corpus luteum

Stage 4: Formation of progesterone in corpus luteum

Stage 5: Corpus luteum shed or maintained

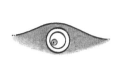

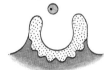

LINING OF UTERUS

Day 1

Day 14

Day 28

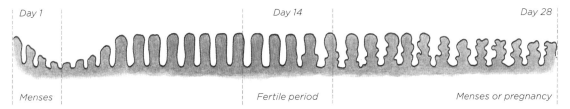

Menses

Fertile period

Menses or pregnancy

Failure to menstruate (amenorrhea): In someone who is menstruating regularly, pregnancy is the first consideration. Other common causes in recent years have been those associated with marked reduction of the fatty tissues of the body, including intensive physical training, extensive dieting, and the anorexia/bulimia syndrome.

Painful menstruation (dysmenorrhea): Menstrual cramps are frequently associated with anxiety and nervous tension. They are most often seen in young women in high-stress situations.

Irregular, excessive, or prolonged menstruation (menorrhagia/ metrorrhagia): There are various reasons, including fibroid (benign) and other tumors, and hormonal imbalances.

Vaginal spotting: This term refers to traces of blood appearing between normal menstrual periods. It may be related to intercourse or the use of tampons, and may represent cervical dysplasia or tumor, so should be investigated with a pelvic examination and a Pap smear test.

Premenstrual syndrome (PMS): This refers to a complex of symptoms occurring before and during menstruation, including irritability, depression, fatigue, headache, and stomachache, with swelling of breasts, abdomen, fingers, and ankles. Some studies suggest that variations in serotonin levels in the body may account for some symptoms; others suggest that low levels of calcium, magnesium, and vitamin B6 may relate to some PMS symptoms.

Menopause: The tapering off of hormone production, mostly between the ages of 40 and 55, can be smooth or bumpy. These hormones influence the blood vessels, and one of the most disturbing symptoms is hot flashes. A more serious consideration is that, with the reduction of natural hormone production, coronary artery disease and osteoporosis may accelerate.

THE MENSTRUAL CYCLE

Illustration showing what happens during a woman's menstrual cycle.

COMPLEMENTARY THERAPIES

Diet and nutrition

Good nutrition is of great importance in maintaining the health of the very complex reproductive system. Evening primrose oil, vitamin B6, calcium, and magnesium are useful supplements.

Exercise

A number of studies indicate that sedentary women who take regular amounts of sustained exercise experience a reduction in PMS symptoms. However, it is important to strike a balance, since very intensive exercise programs can result in the loss of menstrual periods.

Herbal therapy

- Combine sage and blackcurrant leaves and drink as a tea three times a day to relieve the discomfort of hot flashes during the menopause.
- Agnus castus, taken as a decoction or in tincture or pill form on a daily basis, will be of general help for menstrual disorders.
- Combine wild yam, crampbark, pasque flower, marigold, and raspberry leaf and drink as a tea three times a day for period pain.
- Dandelion and parsley act as diuretics.
- Motherwort, skullcap, and passionflower are useful for anxiety and tension.
- Drink raspberry leaf, marigold, nettle, and shepherd's purse as a tea every two to three hours just before and during a period, for heavy bleeding, or for bleeding between periods.

Meditation

Serenity and inner calm are important for hormonal balance and symptom-free menstrual cycles.

Acupressure

Stimulate liver 3 or 13, pericardium 6, spleen 6, or kidney 3 or 6 to provide relief from menstrual symptoms.

Stress management

The value of understanding and dealing with one's life stresses cannot be overemphasized in relation to the reproductive system. Improvement in relationships, work stresses, and other problems will lead to corresponding benefits to the delicate system of communication that governs the menstrual cycle.

Massage

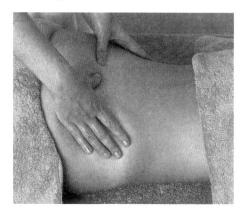

Comfort menstrual pain with slow petrissage in large circles around the sacrum. Begin with palms, and then thumbs close together.

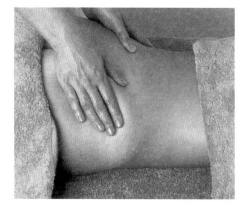

Slowly but rhythmically, circle the thumbs up, out, and back together, gently massaging away the aches that feature in menstruation and PMS.

INFERTILITY

The infertility rate in Western culture is estimated at 10–15 percent, 40–50 percent of which is attributable to the male partner. Most male infertility is related to low sperm motility or low sperm count. The causes of female infertility are much more complex.

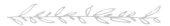

The menstrual cycle is strongly controlled by the pituitary and adrenal glands, and subject to many extraneous influences. For example, severe dieting and/or rigorous exercise resulting in marked loss of fatty tissue can result in loss of menses, hence infertility. Infections and other conditions in the pelvis can cause infertility in women. Some cases of infertility are of psychological origin. The high incidence of pregnancy shortly after adoption supports this view.

A number of other positive correlations have been reported. Alcohol, caffeine, and tobacco have all been implicated in infertility and an increased incidence of spontaneous abortions. Polychlorphenol and lindane have been correlated with infertility in women. These toxins are found in indoor wood and carpet treatments and moth-proofing. Nitrous oxide is associated with increased infertility rates in women. Exposure to solvents, paints, and lead increases infertility in men.

COMPLEMENTARY THERAPIES
Diet and nutrition
Vitamin C, calcium, magnesium, and manganese treatment of the male have been found to increase pregnancy rates in infertile couples. Selenium and zinc are also important to male fertility, and L-carnitine has been found to increase sperm motility where it has been low.

Meditation
The "relaxation response" has been found to decrease anxiety, depression, and fatigue, increase vigor, and result in a pregnancy rate of 34 percent.

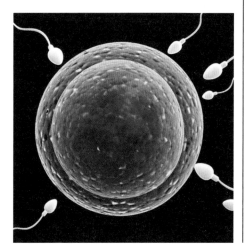

A low sperm count or reduced motility of the sperm are the major causes of male infertility. These can be due to physical, environmental, or psychological factors.

Conventional Therapies

- Hormones
- Psychological counseling
- Surgery for certain tubal and ovarian conditions

SEE ALSO
Symptoms

Therapies

ANAL AND EXTERNAL GENITAL SYMPTOMS

The lower pelvic area is one of considerable local trauma. It contains openings from the digestive tract and the genito-urinary tract, and is also the junction of the trunk with two very active lower extremities.

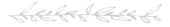

Conventional Therapies

- Steroid, astringent, and antifungal creams and ointments
- Surgery for hemorrhoids, fissure/fistula, local lesions, and hernia

A high-fiber diet, including foods like these, will help promote easy bowel movements.

There are several conditions affecting the lower pelvic region for which complementary therapies are helpful.

Hemorrhoids: These are swollen, inflamed veins that appear at, and just inside, the anal opening, producing pain and sometimes bleeding. They are most common in people whose diets are high in meat and low in fiber, producing hard stools that are difficult to pass. A blood clot can form inside the hemorrhoid. Conventional treatment includes medicated suppositories, sitz baths, and sometimes surgery.

Anal fissure/fistula: An anal fissure is a deep crack in the skin and mucus membrane at the anal opening. It is often a sign of poor nutrition, and secondary infection is common. An anal fistula is a draining sinus connecting the rectal cavity with the outside skin. It is usually a complication of inflammatory bowel disease, and is treated with antibiotics and surgery.

Inflammation of the testicle: There are two types of inflammation, orchitis and epididymitis, which are conventionally treated with antibiotics. Any swelling of the testicle that does not respond completely to therapy should be studied closely for tumor, which is usually completely treatable.

External conditions of the genitals: Most lesions (lumps, sores, etc.) of the external genitals are related in some way to sexual activity, either from injury and irritation or infection of the tissues. If they do not respond promptly to therapy, medical investigation should be carried out to determine the cause.

Inguinal hernia: This is the most common type of hernia, in which part of the intestines protrudes into the canals between the abdominal cavity and the testicles in a male, or in a comparable area in a female (rare). It can be managed by trusses or similar supports, but is most often treated surgically. The situation may be significantly improved by the loss of excess body weight.

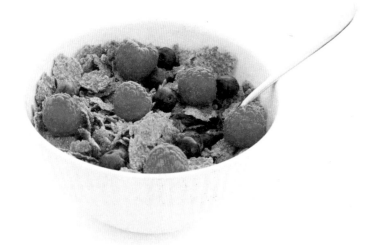

COMPLEMENTARY THERAPIES
Exercise
Regular exercise conditions stomach and back muscles, thus reducing the strain on the bowel.

Diet and nutrition
A diet high in fiber and low in fat will help to prevent hemorrhoids and hernia. Adequate vitamin and mineral supplementation will ensure that the tendency to infection is minimized. Weight control is also important when considering the pelvic organs, which are particularly subject to the forces of gravity.

Hydrotherapy
A sitz bath is a useful therapy, requiring only a small basin to sit in and hot but not scalding water. Incorporate herbs by placing them in a string bag and allowing them to steep in the hot water for a few minutes before settling into the basin. Aloe, common plantain, goldenseal, and witch hazel are especially helpful for hemorrhoids; arnica, borage, coltsfoot, echinacea, and goldenseal are effective against inflammation.

Acupressure

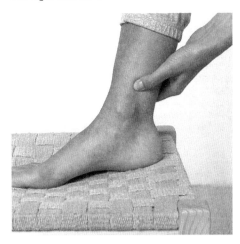

Stimulating spleen 6 aids lower body problems, but do not do this in pregnancy.

Herbal therapy
- Butcher's broom
- Collinsonia
- Cranesbill
- Fluronoids

SEE ALSO
Symptoms
- Infections page 50
- Abdominal pain page 78
- Weight disorders page 146
- Intestinal symptoms page 160

Therapies
- Reflexology page 195
- Homeopathy page 244

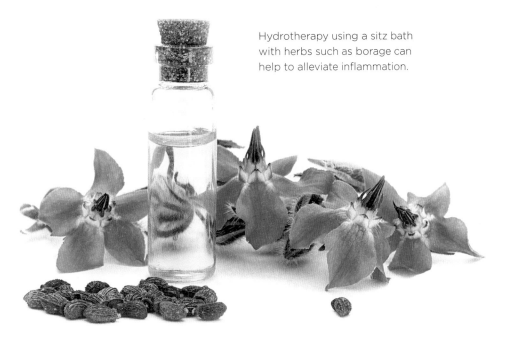

Hydrotherapy using a sitz bath with herbs such as borage can help to alleviate inflammation.

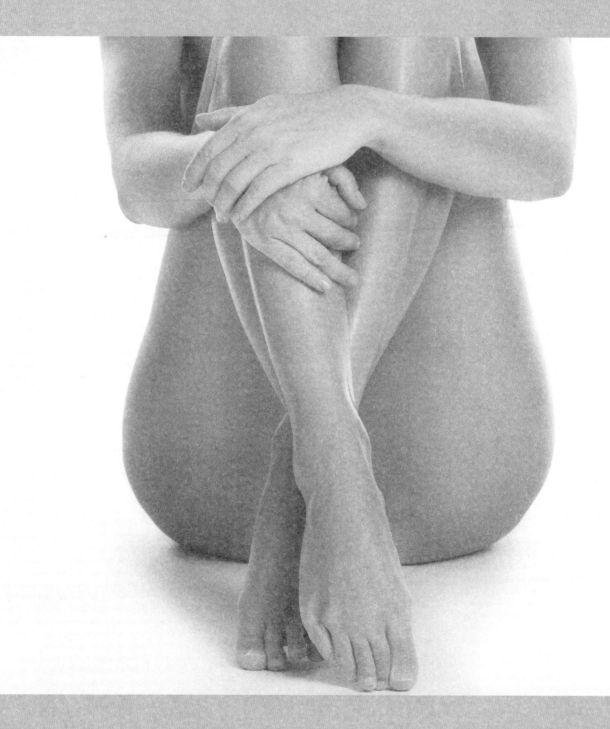

EXTREMITIES & SKIN

JOINT PAIN

Joint pain is a common complaint. It is seldom life-threatening, although it can be the cause of considerable disability. Let us look at some misconceptions about joints and what pain in the neighborhood of a joint signifies.

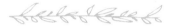

Conventional Therapies

- Anti-inflammatory drugs (some studies show that microscopic blood loss and significant protein loss result from the use of non-steroidal anti-inflammatory drugs—NSAIDs—such as Ibuprofen)

- Pain-relievers

- Physical therapy

- Surgery

A joint is where two (sometimes more) bones come together. Its function is to facilitate pain-free motion of one part of the body in relation to another.

A typical joint is made up of bones; cartilage, a smooth, tough material that covers the ends of the bones; a capsule, an envelope of tissue that creates a closed area called the joint space; and ligaments, tough supporting bands of tissue spanning the joint from bone to bone. Joint pain (also known as arthralgia) is the result of a process going on inside the area defined as the joint.

Three things can cause joint pain.
- Inflammation can come from any process that causes the joint to swell, which often causes it to secrete excess fluid into the joint space.
- Irritation can occur if there is a loose body in the joint space.
- Deterioration occurs most often as a result of injury or aging or both.

Arthritis is inflammation of a joint, but it may have elements of irritation and deterioration as well. The most common types of arthritis are osteoarthritis, rheumatoid arthritis (RA), and gout. What arthritis is not is anything that has its origin outside the joint. Structures near the joints that can cause pain are tendons (tendonitis), bones (osteomyelitis), and muscles (myositis or fibromyalgia).

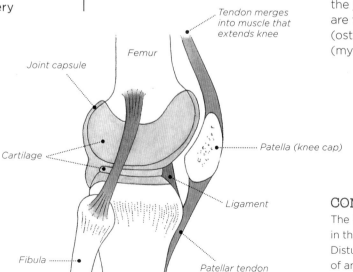

Tendon merges into muscle that extends knee

Femur

Joint capsule

Cartilage

Patella (knee cap)

Ligament

Fibula

Patellar tendon (attached to bone)

Tibia

COMPONENTS OF A JOINT

The knee shows the elements involved in the daily working of a typical joint. Disturbance, damage, or deterioration of any part can cause pain.

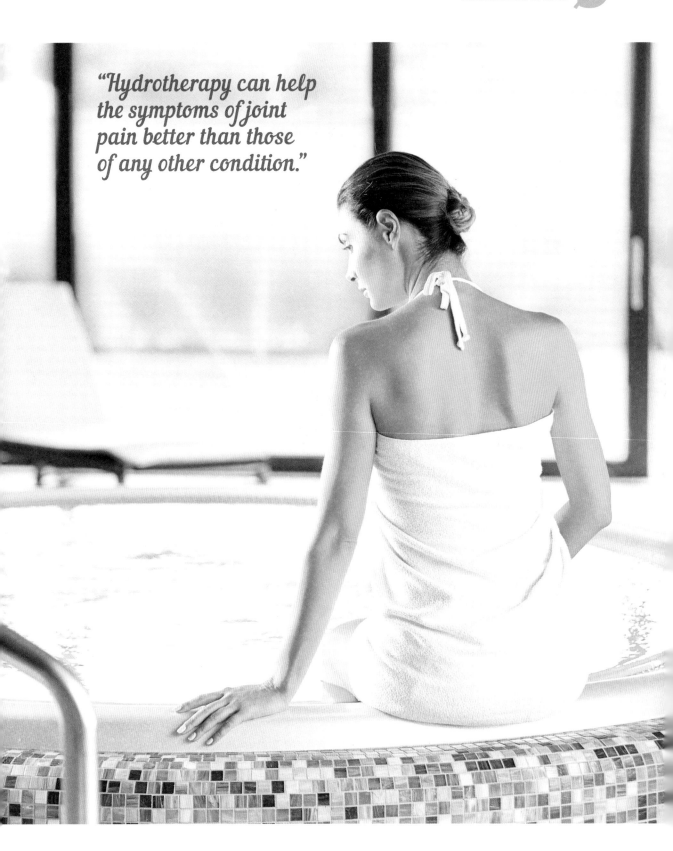

"Hydrotherapy can help the symptoms of joint pain better than those of any other condition."

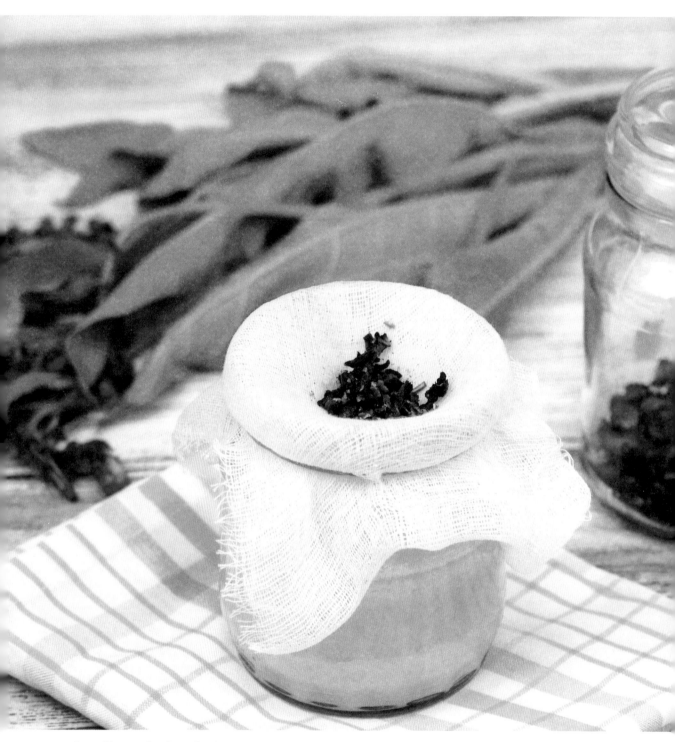

A poultice made of comfrey leaves
applied between gauze soothes
pain and inflammation.

COMPLEMENTARY THERAPIES

Exercise

Stay off work until the painful joint has recovered sufficiently, and any acute inflammation has pretty much subsided. Rest in bed or in a reclining chair, putting the painful area in the most comfortable position. Gradually resume activity when the painful part will tolerate it. Keep in mind that total rest for too long can lead to deconditioning of muscles and prolonged convalescence.

Herbal therapy

- Arnica—first on any list for relieving pain around joints—can be used as a cream or as an ointment.
- Comfrey leaves in a poultice can help with pain and inflammation.
- Equal parts of cayenne pepper (capsicum), mullein leaves, and slippery elm powder, with cider vinegar to dampen the mixture, can be used as a poultice for arthritis and rheumatism.
- Feverfew is useful in general, but specifically for rheumatoid arthritis.
- Ginger has been well-studied and has been proven effective as an anti-inflammatory herb.
- Horsetail can be used as a poultice in arthritis.
- Meadowsweet has pain-relieving properties.

Hydrotherapy

Hydrotherapy is highly recommended for its soothing and healing effects. There are a variety of ways in which to use it effectively for joint pain.

- Warm and hot baths promote the healing of inflammation.
- Swimming will exercise stiffened joints and deconditioned muscles.
- Cold compresses—20 seconds on, 20 seconds off, for five minutes—will help reduce acute swelling.
- Warm compresses and poultices deliver warmth and healing to the affected joint.

Reflexology

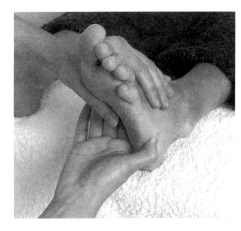

Treat the knee joint from around the indent on the outside of the foot, toward the heel.

Diet and nutrition

Follow your usual nutritious diet, making the amount you eat consistent with your reduced activity. You do not want additional weight to add to the burden of an inflamed joint.

Studies show that some sufferers from rheumatoid arthritis are hypersensitive to certain foods and respond to elimination diets. The most common offending foods include dairy products, cereal, grains, tea, coffee, citrus fruits, red meats, and pork products. Studies of arthritis patients have also shown specific benefits from taking evening primrose oil or blackcurrant oil (gamma linoleic acid), marine lipid oils (EPA and DHA), niacinamide (vitamin B3), and selenium.

Meditation

Relaxation techniques will diminish muscle spasm and pain. Formal studies have shown that relaxation methods are extremely reliable in reducing both pain and inflammation.

SEE ALSO

Symptoms

- Chronic pain page 19
- Back and neck pain page 72
- Weight disorders page 146

Therapies

- Breathing therapy page 190
- Acupressure page 200
- Yoga page 204
- Applied kinesiology page 213
- Stress management page 220
- Music therapy page 224
- Biofeedback page 228
- Homeopathy page 244

CIRCULATORY SYMPTOMS

Symptoms traceable to the arteries and veins of the body can produce great discomfort and disability, sometimes making steady employment impossible. In many people these symptoms tend to become chronic, so it is prudent to begin correcting the problem at the first sign.

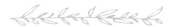

Conventional Therapies

- Topical antibiotic or steroid creams and ointments

- Elastic stockings

- Surgery for varicose veins, arterial blockage, and ulcerations

A number of the symptoms of circulatory problems in the extremities can be helped by complementary therapies. These symptoms relate directly to the adequacy of the blood supply to the affected part, or to any impedance of the blood circulation away from the part.

Pain on exertion: Known as intermittent claudication, this symptom is typical of blockage of an artery or arteries leading to the extremities. It is the same process that produces chest pain by blocking the coronary arteries. If it occurs in the legs, pain appears consistently after a certain amount of exertion and gradually goes away when the exertion ceases. The conventional treatment of this process is almost entirely surgical, consisting of the removal of the blocked segment of artery and its substitution by a length of vein.

Swelling: Circulatory problems can produce swelling (edema) of the hands or feet by changing the pressure gradients in the extremities and forcing fluid into the soft tissues. However, several other conditions regularly cause swelling of hands and especially feet, including heart failure, liver failure, kidney failure, and low serum protein. Conventional therapy treats the primary cause of the swelling.

Redness and blanching: In cases of arterial blockage, the extremity may blanch when elevated and redden when lowered.

Ulceration: When either arterial or venous circulation is poor, the skin may break down, especially over pressure points like the ankle, and ulcers form.

Varicose veins: The veins are equipped with internal valves that keep the blood, which is being pushed toward the heart, from sliding back in the opposite direction. In the legs, the valves, together with the action of the leg muscles, prevent blood going back toward the foot. When the pressure in a vein rises, a valve may be overcome, causing a further pressure rise. Over time, the vein distends, becoming varicose. The main causes of the increased pressure are being overweight, pregnancy, and anything else causing congestion of the pelvic structures, thus impeding venous flow upward. Conventional treatment of varicose veins includes elastic stockings and surgery.

"Aches and pains in the hands, legs, and feet are often the result of poor circulation of blood in those areas."

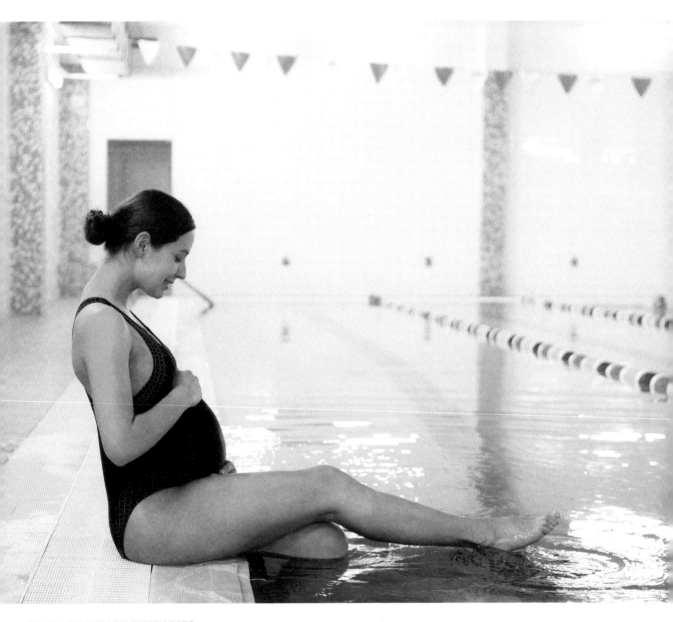

COMPLEMENTARY THERAPIES
Exercise

It is a mistake to conclude that exercise is bad because it produces some symptoms in arterial disease in the legs. On the contrary, exercise promotes the development of collateral channels around arterial blocks when it is carried out on a regular basis. Don't push the exercise to the point of significant pain, but do it regularly. Walking on level ground and swimming are the best kinds of exercise for circulatory problems. They also keep muscles in tone and control weight.

Standing for long periods, at work for example, can increase susceptibility to varicose veins, so avoid standing still if possible or exercise your calf muscles by moving your feet up and down for a few minutes at regular intervals.

Good diet and exercise can ward off varicose veins due to increased pressure in pregnancy.

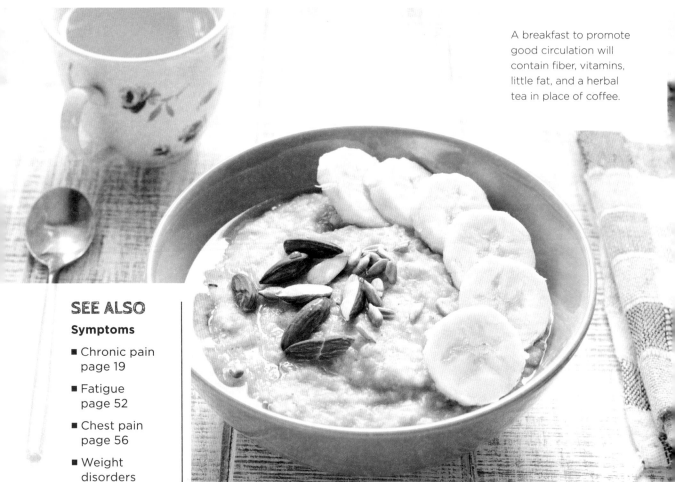

A breakfast to promote good circulation will contain fiber, vitamins, little fat, and a herbal tea in place of coffee.

Acupressure

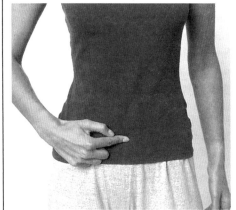

Massaging the body's energy center, about two fingers' width below the navel, tones circulation.

Diet and nutrition

Since the process that produces arterial obstruction in the extremities is the same as that in the coronary arteries of the heart, the same criteria apply. See Chest Pain on page 56; and Diet and Nutrition on page 175 for details of optimal diet programs.

Weight control is very important for problems affecting veins; they are roughly proportional to the degree of excess weight present.

SOFT TISSUE SYMPTOMS

There are several common problems, other than arthritis, that afflict the soft tissues of the body. These are important, particularly because pain and interference with function often result.

The symptoms that occur in the extremities, other than trouble in the joints (arthritis), can arise from outside injury or as a result of other processes within the body.

Aches and pains: This nonspecific complaint has also been called rheumatism in times past. It refers to discomfort not strictly related to any joint but with symptoms like those of arthritis. Specialists may call it periarthritis, fibrositis, fasciitis, and non-articular rheumatism. Localized forms may be labeled tendonitis at the wrist or epicondylitis. This discomfort can arise from muscles, tendons, ligaments, or fascia (the heavy sheet of tissue covering muscle). It is an inflammatory condition and overuse of the affected part is at the root of a high proportion of cases. Conventional treatment includes pain-relievers, anti-inflammatory drugs, and physical therapy.

Symptoms related to nerve supply: These include numbness and tingling, pain, and sensations of heat or cold. The best-known conditions are carpal tunnel syndrome and thoracic outlet syndrome, and there are a few others that are similar. These have been shown to be caused by combinations of overuse, being overweight, poor diet, and poor posture. The symptoms are caused by pressure on nerve trunks as they traverse the extremity. People with these symptoms often require surgery to relieve the offending pressure.

Soft tissue injuries: In this category, fall bruises, strains, and sprains, which are conventionally treated with pain-relieving drugs, rest, and splinting.

Conventional Therapies

- Pain-relieving drugs
- Anti-inflammatory drugs
- Physical therapy
- Rest and splinting
- Surgery

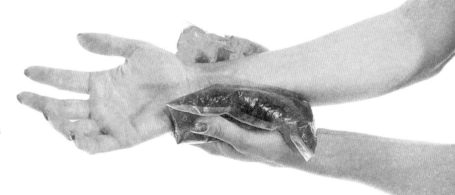

Treat a sprain immediately with a gelatin cold pack or a compress of ice wrapped in a thin towel. Leave for 30 minutes and repeat several times a day.

SEE ALSO

Symptoms

- Back and neck pain page 72
- Joint pain page 94
- Weight disorders page 146

Therapies

- Reflexology page 195
- Homeopathy page 244

Yoga helps increase muscle strength and flexibility, both of which play a part in avoiding injury.

COMPLEMENTARY THERAPIES
Massage

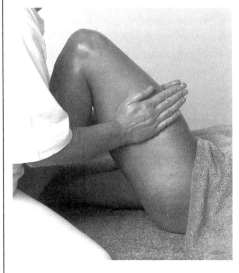

To relax and restore overworked front of thigh muscles after exercise, apply oil and massage with your palms in slow, rhythmic strokes, working more strongly toward the heart.

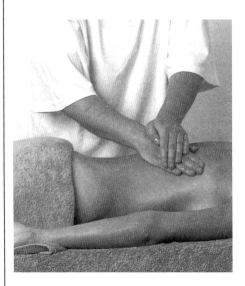

Circular "ironing" up each side of the back is beneficial for soothing and refreshing aching muscles. Do not apply pressure to the spinal cord or to any inflamed or newly bruised areas.

Diet and nutrition

- Vitamin B6 in doses of 100–200mg per day is effective in a high proportion of cases of carpal tunnel syndrome, on the pain threshold as well as on controlling inflammation.
- Weight control is a critical factor in thoracic outlet syndrome, which involves pressure on the nerves at the shoulder, and may be a factor in other situations affecting soft tissues.

Hydrotherapy

- Cold compresses are effective for acute sprains. They minimize swelling and bleeding into the tissues.
- Warm baths are helpful in all cases of extremity discomfort, both for general relaxation and for the relief of local stiffness and pain.
- Whirlpool baths are effective for local inflammation, as they stimulate the circulation, causing irritating waste products to be carried away from injured tissues.

Alexander technique

Proper alignment of the body is important in the dynamics of thoracic outlet syndrome, and this technique can help achieve it.

Exercise

The best prevention of strains and sprains is a consistent program of conditioning through exercise, which makes muscles strong and tends to prevent problems like hypertension and hyperflexion, i.e. stretching and bending joints and muscles too far. Activities in the workplace should be organized so that repetitive tasks alternate with other jobs that do not place stress on the same structures. This lessens the tendency to carpal tunnel syndrome, thoracic outlet syndrome, and the condition known as "overuse" or repetitive strain injury.

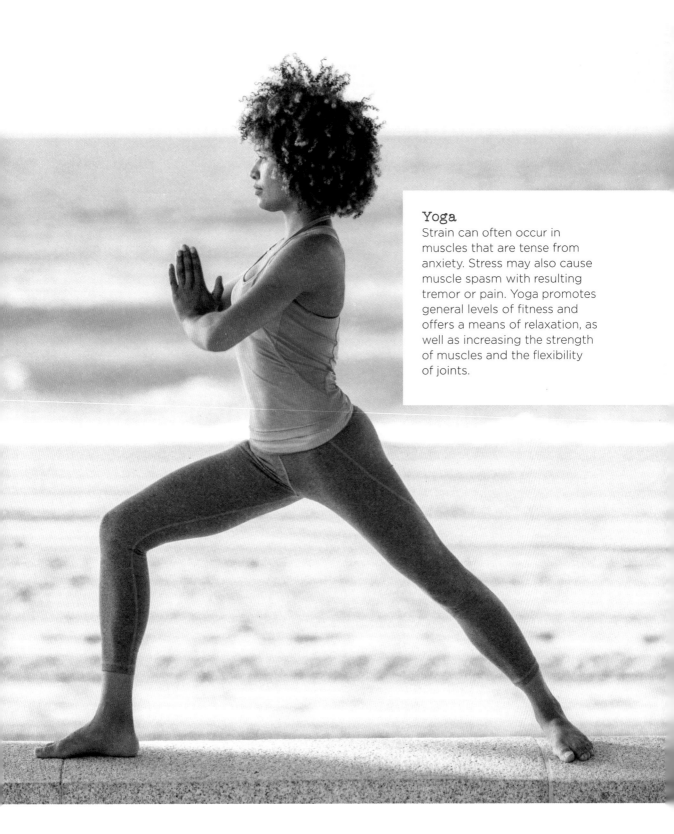

Yoga

Strain can often occur in muscles that are tense from anxiety. Stress may also cause muscle spasm with resulting tremor or pain. Yoga promotes general levels of fitness and offers a means of relaxation, as well as increasing the strength of muscles and the flexibility of joints.

SKIN SYMPTOMS

The skin is considered a vital organ, since the functional loss of more than a certain percentage of it results in death. With the great advances in massive burn therapy in the past few decades, people can now survive with only 10–25 percent of their skin intact.

Conventional Therapies

- Topical applications and dressings

- Topical drugs, especially steroids

- Systemic drugs, largely to suppress symptoms (steroids have proved dangerous because of the seriousness of the side-effects and the temptation to long-term use)

- Surgery

The skin is a complex membranous envelope composed of the outer skin, the hair, nails, and subcutaneous tissue. It is continuous with the mucus membrane lining the gastrointestinal and respiratory tracts, which facilitates the transfer of nutrients from food and oxygen from the air to their final destination in the body's cells.

The skin is a very versatile organ. It protects against physical, chemical, and microbial injury and perceives a wide variety of noxious stimuli. It helps to regulate the body temperature and monitors the flow of water and salts leaving the body.

It also provides an elastic covering that accommodates the movements of the underlying structures.

The skin's health depends on the maintenance of a number of delicate balances, such as the production of oil and sweat, which are determined by a host of interacting factors throughout the body.

There are very many ways in which the skin can deviate from its usual pattern of functioning.

Abscess: This is a localized area of inflammation under the skin that heals by gradually forming a firm nodule containing pus. The only way it can be resolved is by incision and drainage.

THE SKIN
The skin performs vital protective, perceptive, and temperature and fluid control functions.

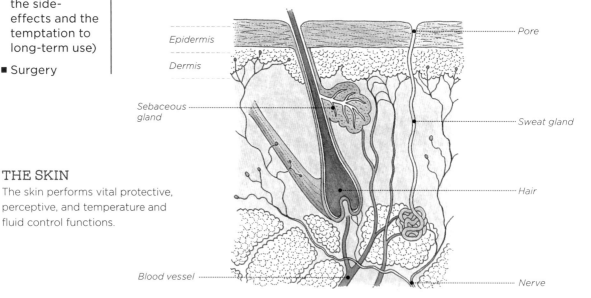

Epidermis

Dermis

Sebaceous gland

Blood vessel

Pore

Sweat gland

Hair

Nerve

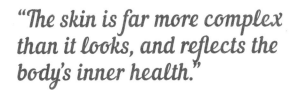

"The skin is far more complex than it looks, and reflects the body's inner health."

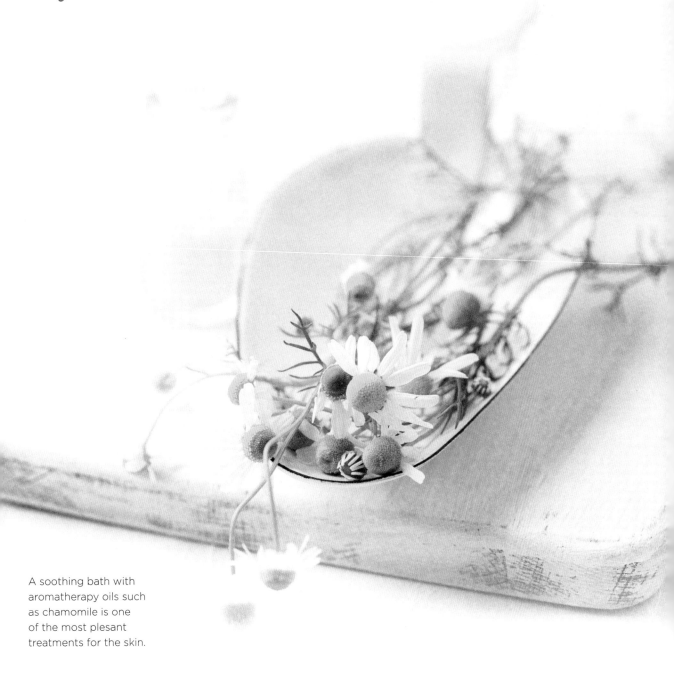

A soothing bath with aromatherapy oils such as chamomile is one of the most plesant treatments for the skin.

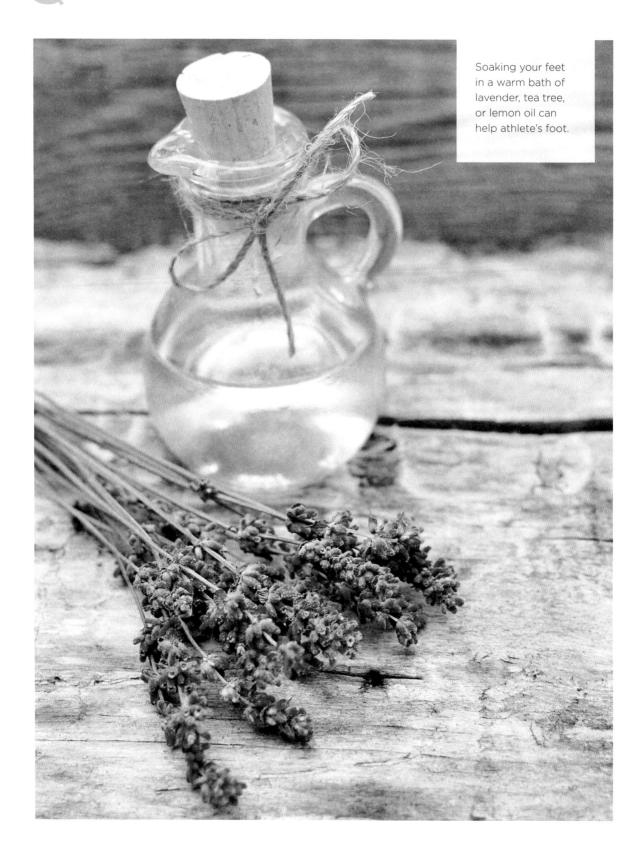

Soaking your feet in a warm bath of lavender, tea tree, or lemon oil can help athlete's foot.

Acne: This well-known affliction of adolescence begins as inflammation around a hair follicle, usually aggravated by attempts to remove it manually, with secondary infection resulting. Acne is seen to some degree in about 80 percent of teenagers. It is caused primarily by the effect of emerging sex hormones on the hair/sebaceous gland complex, but it is known to be intensified by the consumption of a diet high in fats and fried foods. It is treated variously by cleansing and scrubbing the skin and the use of antibacterial and anti-inflammatory drugs. Dermabrasion (peeling off the outer layer of skin) has been used in advanced cases.

Athlete's foot and ringworm: These are the most common fungus infections of the skin. Athlete's foot usually affects the skin between the toes, but may become more extensive. It is usually acquired in locker rooms and group shower rooms that are not carefully cleaned. Ringworm infections of the body, nails, and scalp have nothing to do with worms, but are also fungal infections, named after their typical circular pattern. There are now specific antifungal agents, such as sulconazole, that are effective and have only a few mild local side-effects.

Body odor: The most noticeable odors emanate from the sweat glands of the armpit, groin, and feet. Some people do not find body odors offensive, but beyond a point most people do. Regular bathing not only minimizes this problem, but it is better for the skin as well, since it removes debris and excreted salts from the surface of the skin.

Boils and carbuncles: Boils (furuncles) are inflammatory nodules around hair follicles caused by bacterial infection. They form a liquid center from which pus eventually escapes, either spontaneously or after incision. A carbuncle occurs when a group of infected follicles coalesce to form an extensive pocket of infection. Incision and drainage is the preferred treatment, and scarring usually results.

Burn injuries: These range from trivial to lethal. In recent years, large burn treatment centers have developed and their work has materially improved the chances of recovery for victims of extensive burns. We tend to think of burns as thermal injuries, but electrical, chemical, and radioactive agents produce the same effects, i.e. the denaturing of cell protein. Fire victims may also suffer from burns of the respiratory tract, and extensive burns may be complicated by kidney failure. Less serious burns are treated with applications of salves and lotions, and medication to combat pain.

Candida: This is the name of a yeast organism that can invade tissues, especially in the vagina and the gastrointestinal tract. Though it is an organism, not a symptom, people are often told they "have Candida," so it sounds like "having flu." Yeast organisms are found in the intestinal tract of a high percentage of the general public, possibly due to the prevalence of yeast-containing foods, such as bread and beer, ingested over many generations. Under certain conditions their numbers increase in the body, overwhelming the host defenses and producing illness. Many of the effects are believed to be allergic in nature. There is evidence that antibiotics, by killing off many of the normal bacterial microflora of the intestinal tract, pave the way for colonization by Candida. The intestine is believed to be the reservoir for Candida that infects the mouth and vagina. Candidiasis is a prominent feature of AIDS, and any person under immunosuppression with steroids is at increased risk of Candida infection. Diabetics are also unduly susceptible. Candida is conventionally treated by a variety of drugs, many of which have side-effects.

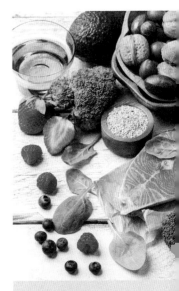

Eat MORE

- Vegetables, vegetable oils, and oily fish such as tuna and mackerel.

Eat LESS

- Dairy products, the most common food allergens.

- Animal fats, sugars, and salts.

- Processed food, and foods with additives and preservatives.

"A tendency to eczema (chronic dermatitis) is lifelong and there is as yet no cure, but a wide range of natural approaches can help."

Herbal teas that can provide relief from a variety of skin conditions include dandelion (below), red clover, borage, burdock, nettle, comfrey, and marigold.

Cellulite: This is a term for the fatty deposits that cause "orange-peel" skin on the buttocks and thighs. It may concern those who have it, but is of no medical significance. There is no recognized conventional therapy at present.

Cold sores: These are caused by the *Herpes simplex* virus, which appears to enter tissues early in life and lie dormant until much later, when small vesicles filled with clear fluid emerge on the skin or mucus membranes, surrounded by an inflamed base. This emergence may occur in the context of overexposure to the sun, respiratory or other infections, or emotional stress. The conventional treatment is nonspecific (soothing ointments and so on).

Cysts: These are firm, fluid-filled nodules. The most common cyst of the skin is the sebaceous cyst or wen, which results from blockage of the duct leading from a sebaceous gland to the surface, producing a nodule that can be tender or unsightly. The conventional treatment for cysts is excision.

Dermatitis: A chronic superficial inflammation of the skin, dermatitis features redness, oozing, crusting, scaling, and sometimes vesicle formation. It constitutes more than half of all skin conditions. Eczema is another name for chronic dermatitis. It falls into several classifications.

Contact dermatitis is inflammation produced by substances coming in contact with the skin. Sensitivity may follow repeated exposure (as in poison ivy). Conventional treatment is by removal of the offending agent and the use of medications to suppress the reaction and relieve the symptoms. Atopic dermatitis is chronic, itchy, superficial inflammation in people with personal or family histories of allergic disorders, such as hay fever or asthma. Treatment may involve allergy testing and desensitization. Seborrheic dermatitis is chronic, itchy inflammation with redness and scaling, found in conjunction with acne, dandruff, and other oily skin conditions. Neuro-dermatitis is chronic inflammation with thick, dry, flaking patches and intense itching. It is said to have a strong psychological component. The itching and skin changes are made worse by scratching, which is increased by stress and tension. There are other varieties, but the above are the most usual.

Infestations: Scabies and lice are the most common. Both start in the home with poor hygiene, and then break out in places such as schools, spreading to a whole group of people together. Treatment is by bathing and cleaning

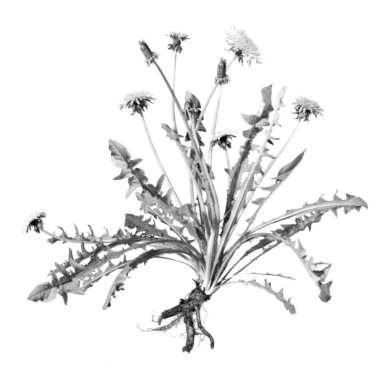

the environment, plus specific medications; any good pharmacist will know what is currently safest and most effective.

Itching: This is an important symptom of skin inflammation. It is sometimes found in jaundice and kidney failure. See the comments on the individual conditions for information.

Rashes: These occur in a great variety of situations, some of which have been described above. See the individual conditions discussed.

Shingles: This is a condition in which the *Herpes zoster* virus infects the roots of a peripheral nerve anywhere in the body. The effects spread along the course of the nerve, producing considerable pain in the area and the eruption of clumps of encrusted vesicles. The crusts fall off within a couple of weeks; the pain may last days or many months. Conventional treatment includes pain-relieving drugs and local anesthetics; steroids have been injected into the painful areas with variable results.

Tumors: These include several types of cancerous lesions, which are usually controlled by local excision, although there is a strong tendency to local recurrence. Skin cancer is promoted by overexposure to the sun's rays, especially in fair-skinned people, and protective measures should be taken by everybody when going out in the sun.

COMPLEMENTARY THERAPIES
Herbal therapy

- Burdock, chickweed, comfrey, and marigold, as compresses or ointment, will soothe irritated skin.
- Burdock, cleavers, dandelion, echinacea, red clover, and yellow dock can be drunk as a tea for acne.
- Chickweed, elderflower, and marigold, combined in equal parts and used as a facial steam, may help acne.
- Red clover, borage, burdock root, and nettles will soothe inflamed skin.

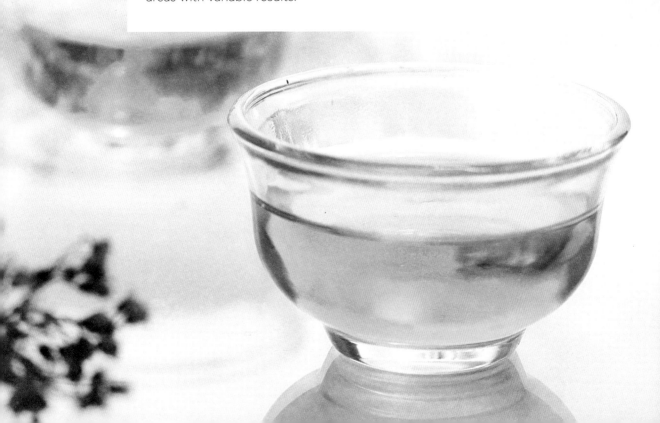

SEE ALSO

Symptoms

- Infections page 50
- Anxiety and panic page 130
- Eating disorders page 142
- Jaundice page 156
- Symptoms relating to immune function page 166
- Aging page 170

Therapies

- Reflexology page 195
- Imagery page 218
- Homeopathy page 244

Reflexology

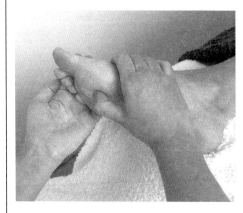

Stimulating the thymus and other gland reflexes benefits skin quality, elasticity, and moisture balance. The pituitary reflex is especially useful for treating acne.

Massage

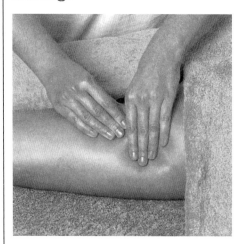

Firmly kneading the back of the thighs combats cellulite by enhancing cellular functioning.

Stress management

In many instances, dermatitis is a reflection of turmoil in everyday life. It is well to look at one's personal relationships at home and at work, to see if they can be conducted more gently, fairly, and lovingly.

Meditation

Your preferred meditation technique will be very helpful in coping with the often unpleasant symptoms of dermatitis, where great calmness of spirit is beneficial. Regular practice of meditation helps to reach the deeper causes of problems, soothing them and healing them, as well as relieving the tension aroused by persistent irritation.

Aromatherapy

- Put five drops each of lemon, cypress, and juniper oils in 2oz (60g) water, mix well, and bathe the area affected by acne several times a day. At night, use the same essences in a carrier oil.
- Dab pure lavender oil every hour onto the affected skin during an acute attack of eczema.
- Chamomile, lavender, and geranium oils used in the bathtub, as a compress, or in a carrier oil for massage will help eczema. (Do not massage over areas of broken skin.)
- Lavender, tea tree, or lemon oils in a warm foot bath will help athlete's foot.
- Use ten drops each of lavender and tea tree oils and five drops of geranium oil in a carrier oil for ringworm. Apply it with cotton balls at regular intervals to the affected area.
- Mix four to six drops each of bergamot, eucalyptus, and tea tree oils in 2oz (60g) of a carrier oil and apply regularly to cold sores.
- Massage a blend of six drops of rosemary or tea tree oil, five drops of eucalyptus or geranium oil, and six drops of lavender oil in 2oz (60g) of carrier oil into the scalp to treat head lice. Wrap the hair in a towel or plastic wrap for up to two hours, then comb through and shampoo thoroughly. Repeat daily as necessary.

Diet and nutrition

A healthy nutritional program is just as important for the skin as it is for other, less visible body tissues. The skin requires a balance to assure that it is thick enough, moist enough, elastic enough, and so on. Such a balance derives in large measure from the maintenance of the body's many overall balances and nutrition plays a major role. Specifically, adequate amounts of the following are especially beneficial to the skin.

- Vitamins A, B-complex, and E
- Marine lipids obtained from fish oils
- Evening primrose oil or other sources of gamma-linolenic acid
- Zinc, selenium, and magnesium
- Lysine (to treat *Herpes simplex*)

Hydrotherapy

Short warm baths are useful for cleansing debris from inflamed or caked skin. Pat dry and apply therapeutic oils as indicated by the condition.

The Dead Sea resorts between Israel and Jordan have an unequalled reputation for treating skin conditions. At 1,300ft (400m) below sea level, the atmosphere naturally filters out the harmful rays and leaves only the beneficial UVA and UVB rays. This, coupled with bathing in the Dead Sea itself and the mud around it—both high in minerals good for skin nourishment—provides the almost perfect skin treatment.

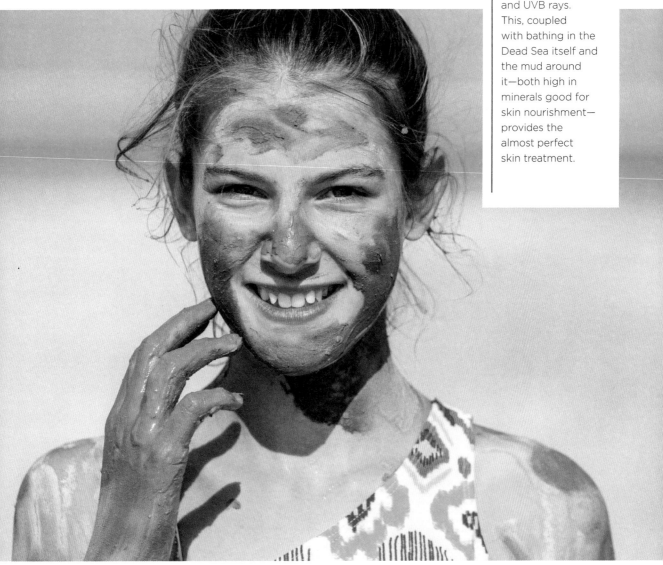

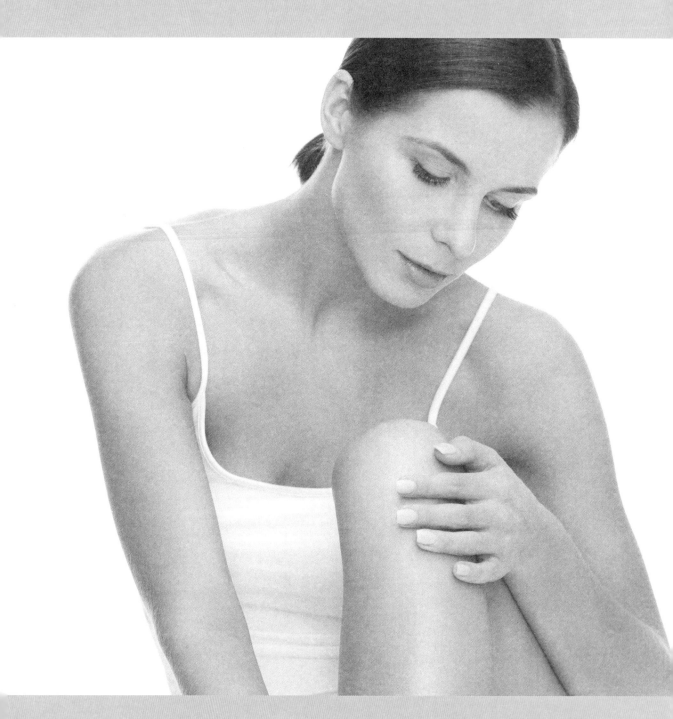

NERVOUS SYSTEM

SEIZURES

A seizure (i.e. convulsion, fit) occurs when there is a sudden disorderly electrical discharge of nerve cells in the brain. This sends unusual signals through the system, resulting in distinct patterns that can be recognized as seizures. A person with recurring seizures is said to have epilepsy or seizure disorder.

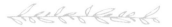

Gluten-free foods like these, the remedy for celiac disease, limit seizures in child sufferers who also have epilepsy.

Seizures are classified into the following groups, according to how they present themselves.

Grand mal: This is the best-known type of seizure. It is a dramatic generalized convulsion. There is a sudden loss of consciousness with the patient falling to the ground, preceded in about half the cases by an aura (some sensation that indicates what is to come) and followed—in order—by a spasm of all the muscles, a series of violent, jerking movements of the whole body, and then a deep coma. The person awakes in a confused state, only to fall into a deep sleep lasting for several hours. There may be other symptoms or some variations in the above description.

Petit mal: In contrast, these spells are so brief that they may be overlooked by others. The person loses consciousness but as a rule does not fall. Remaining motionless, staring into space, and failing to respond to conversation comprise the typical

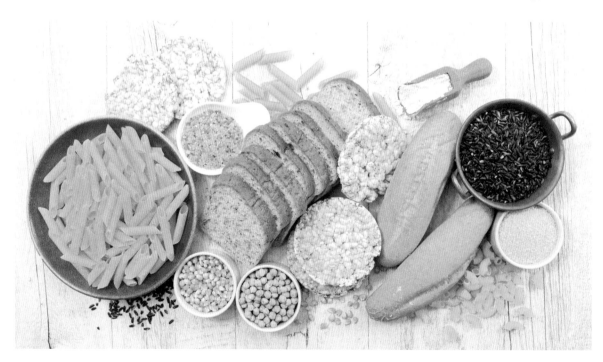

picture of this type of seizure. After 2–15 seconds, the person abruptly regains consciousness and resumes the activity that was interrupted by the seizure.

Psychomotor: This type differs from those above in the following ways.

- An aura, if present, may be a complex hallucination or perceptual illusion.
- The duration may be from seconds to a number of days.
- Rather than amnesia for the period of the seizure, the person may have something like a dream experience; things seem far away or a sense of déjà vu may occur.
- To others, the person appears to be behaving automatically, with a few repetitive movements of the face or of the extremities.

Flickering illuminations and screens, and strobe lights in particular, have been known to cause seizures. Other causes can be classified in several ways: vascular problems—especially thrombosis or embolism; tumors—especially those close to the motor cortex; trauma—usually six months to two years after a head injury; infections—including brain abscess and encephalitis; and degenerative diseases—rare, but including multiple sclerosis.

COMPLEMENTARY THERAPIES
Diet and nutrition
Some studies point to magnesium deficiency as predisposing to seizures. Supplementation with magnesium will complement any other control measures being used. Blood and tissue levels of manganese, another trace mineral, have also been found to correlate with the incidence of seizures, especially where their frequency is great. Severe deficiencies in vitamin B6 are also known to be connected with the incidence of seizures.

All the dietary measures that lead to optimal nutrition are particularly applicable to seizure prevention, because they will ensure that the circulation of blood to all parts of the brain is maximized. A gluten-free diet has been shown to be effective in reducing seizure frequency in children with epilepsy. Deficiencies of several nutrients have been linked to the use of anticonvulsant drugs, including folate, thiamine, vitamin B12, vitamin D, and vitamin E. Restoration of normal levels through supplementation may lead to a reduction in seizure frequency.

Biofeedback
A number of studies have shown that biofeedback training is effective in reducing the frequency of seizures by as much as 35 percent. This requires the services of an experienced trainer, but the method enables the person to assume full control of the exercises after the completion of training.

Acupressure
If you are near a person with a seizure, remain calm. Remove furniture so that the person is in a clear space. Place a folded handkerchief between the upper and lower teeth, loosen the clothing, and place a wet towel on the head. When the person is quiet, do the following. Press the bladder meridian along the spine, governing vessels 14 and 26, bladder 60, and CV 12. Press hard on the Achilles tendon and then pinch the big toe with your thumb and index finger. Finally, press hard on the palms.

Meditation
Relaxation techniques can help to reduce the frequency and even the severity of seizures, and learning how to meditate can be especially beneficial.

Conventional Therapies

- Anticonvulsant drugs
- Surgery

SEE ALSO

MENTAL SYMPTOMS

The interpretation of the signs and symptoms of mental illness is quite difficult. This is partly because there are many shades of gray between what is considered "normal" and "abnormal." Who among us has not felt a bit "crazy" when we were very tired and stressed, and everybody else in the vicinity was running around noisily?

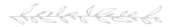

Conventional Therapies

- Drugs (mood-altering, tranquilizing, and sedative)

- Institutional care (mental hospitals and community care homes)

- Home care (visiting nurse and volunteer services)

In that circumstance we may lose our concentration, forget what we were thinking just a moment ago, or feel that everybody is ganging up on us. In that moment we could be classified as mentally ill, but the moment passes when we go outside for a breath of air to get away from the confusion, and we feel "normal" again. A truly mentally ill person will not be able to regain balance in a short space of time and will become dysfunctional as the state of being overwhelmed continues. That is when something needs to happen to turn things around.

In addition to the acute situation described above, there are many other aspects of mental functioning, including prevention of illness, the recognition of mild symptoms, management of chronic symptoms, and mental deterioration.

First, there are many symptoms to consider. Each may appear in any degree from mild to severe. Mild symptoms do not constitute mental illness; severe degrees may do so. Here are a few of the symptoms.

Attention disorders: In their mildest form, these manifest themselves as momentary "absence" or inattention, such as you might experience when you are very tired and cannot keep track of what you are doing. When prolonged, this could appear as failure to comprehend a simple instruction or thought expressed by another person. In most instances this clears up when you "pull yourself together" or decide to get some rest.

Mood and affect disorders: When you are tired or stressed, you may become either "wired up" or "down in the dumps," out of proportion to what is going on at the time. It probably sorts itself out after a good nap or a period

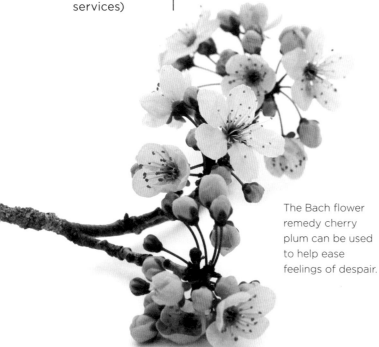

The Bach flower remedy cherry plum can be used to help ease feelings of despair.

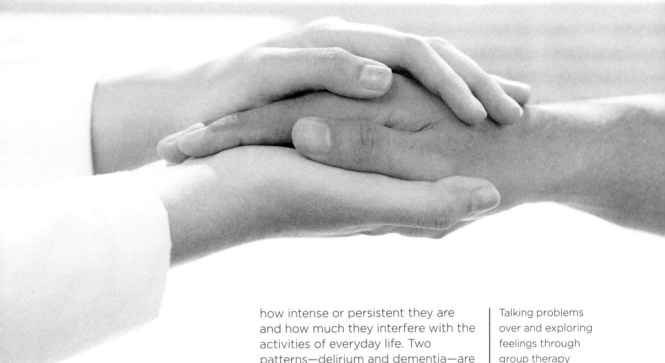

how intense or persistent they are and how much they interfere with the activities of everyday life. Two patterns—delirium and dementia—are worthy of brief mention here.

Delirium: This is an acute condition, occurring most often in the context of infection, intoxication with any of a variety of toxins, or in the withdrawal stage of the use of substances like alcohol or drugs. Its features include mental clouding and diminished attention; hallucinations and/or delusions; excessive motor activity; mood/affect disorders; autonomic overactivity (fever, sweating, and rapid heart action). The appearance of these symptoms is a signal to seek medical attention.

Dementia: This term refers to a combination of symptoms that is chronic, progressive, and degenerative. It is typically gradual in onset, the earliest manifestations being very subtle deviations from the norm. Dementia has a multitude of settings and causes, including "cause unknown." Symptoms, as they become more definable, include gradual loss of insight, orientation, and memory; impairment of mental activity in the areas of calculation and abstract thought; alteration of

Talking problems over and exploring feelings through group therapy or individual counseling can bring support and a sense of relief.

of relaxation. If the mood is prolonged or the pattern becomes entrenched, it may assume the proportions of a problem. One's affect is the outward expression of emotion or mood. A person who characteristically under-expresses emotion is said to have a bland or flat affect. This can be significant when combined with other symptoms.

Thought disorders: These can be divided as follows.

- Hallucinations and illusions are disorders of perception.
- Delusions are false or erroneous beliefs.
- Paranoia is an example of a false interpretation of reality.

When various symptoms occur in combination, significant patterns, or syndromes, can sometimes be recognized. There are far too many such syndromes to be described here. The important thing is to recognize the above tendencies in yourself or in friends or loved ones, and to estimate

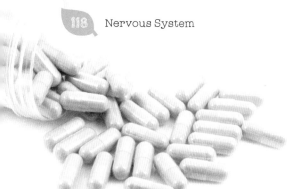

The use of high doses of certain vitamins is a recognized but controversial approach to the treatment of mental dysfunction.

behavior in the areas of attitudes, general bearing, stream of thought, attentiveness, personal hygiene, mood, etc. The example of dementia that has received the most attention in recent years is Alzheimer's disease, which continues to undergo intensive study, with few definitive results.

COMPLEMENTARY THERAPIES
Diet and nutrition

The effect of nutrition on mental functioning is a subject over which controversy has flourished in the past 30 years. One of the focal points of this discussion is what Professor Linus Pauling called "orthomolecular medicine and psychiatry." Pauling and others who followed in his footsteps have demonstrated that various forms of mental dysfunction improve significantly during and after the use of certain vitamins in much higher amounts than are listed in the recommended dietary allowances (RDA). These demonstrations have resulted in the concept of optimal nutrition for optimal health and have led to a well-recognized specialty of nutritional medicine. This high-dose vitamin usage is sometimes called megavitamin therapy, especially by its critics.

Meditation trains you to focus on an inner haven where negative thoughts cannot enter.

Orthomolecular medicine (including psychiatry) is based on the idea that the right molecule (found in a vitamin) can supply a missing ingredient in a misbehaving cell of the nervous system, causing that cell to resume its normal functioning. It was found that the usual RDA-level doses of several vitamins did not produce this result, but that doses many times higher did so. The conclusion was that balance and stability, in the nervous system particularly, are enhanced by the regular use of higher doses of certain vitamins, in particular those of the B group and vitamin C.

Please refer to Diet and Nutrition in the therapy section for additional details of optimal nutrition.

Stress management

Lifestyle issues, such as interpersonal relationships and one's job situation, can have a direct bearing on mental stability. It is as well to keep these influences in mind at all times, but especially when you are feeling overwhelmed or off-balance.

Bach flower remedies

This therapy is particularly suited to the management of mental attitudes and conditions. The following remedies have been found to be effective.
- Agrimony (mental distress)
- Cherry plum (deep despair)
- Scleranthus (indecision and uncertainty)

Exercise

Exercise of a kind that you enjoy (e.g. swimming, cycling, walking, playing sport) can be an excellent antidote to milder mental symptoms and the physical symptoms that may accompany them, by raising energy levels and channeling attention elsewhere. Again, it is wise to develop this habit on a regular basis before symptoms strike.

"Feelings of worry and dejection are universal, but vary in intensity and can become overwhelming."

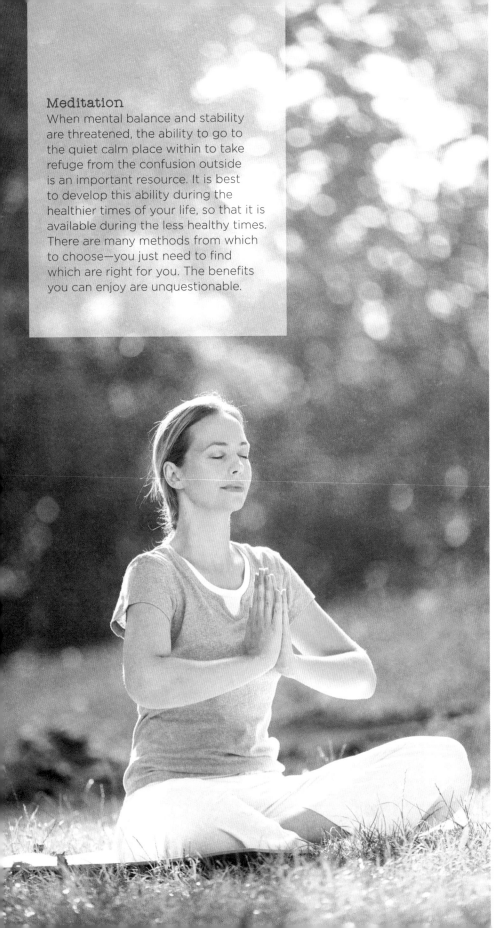

Meditation

When mental balance and stability are threatened, the ability to go to the quiet calm place within to take refuge from the confusion outside is an important resource. It is best to develop this ability during the healthier times of your life, so that it is available during the less healthy times. There are many methods from which to choose—you just need to find which are right for you. The benefits you can enjoy are unquestionable.

WEAKNESS AND PARALYSIS

There is a wide spectrum of conditions in which there is loss of strength or vital energy. These conditions produce effects ranging from slight weakness to disabling paralysis.

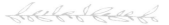

Conventional Therapies

- Treatment of pain

- Physical therapy

- Surgery

- Social intervention in severe situations

SEE ALSO

Symptoms

- Flu symptoms page 48

- Infections page 50

- Fatigue page 52

Therapies

- Diet and nutrition page 175

- Imagery page 218

- Group therapy page 223

The following commonly encountered symptoms can be appropriately managed with a variety of complementary therapies.

Weakness: This may be separated into two categories. The first is generalized weakness, which may be the result of tiredness or excessive stress, or may be one aspect of a virus infection, such as flu. Weakness may be conspicuous in chronic fatigue syndrome. It is also quite usual in acute shock from whatever cause. The second category is localized weakness, which may be a specific neurological sign of inflammation of, or pressure on, a nerve or group of nerves. It may be associated with altered sensation, such as numbness, tingling, or a hot/cold sensation.

Localized paralysis: This may be an initial symptom or a progression from local weakness. It is also due to some process affecting a single nerve or nerve group. It can occur in any part of the body and can affect speech, vision, or movement. In multiple sclerosis there is patchy involvement of the covering of individual nerves, resulting in scattered areas of local paralysis.

Hemiparesis: This is paralysis of one side of the body, usually as a result of interference with the circulation of blood to a part of the brain. It is usually referred to as a stroke. Speech may be impaired if the dominant cerebral hemisphere is affected. Personality change may occur as a result, depending in part on the degree of impairment that has been suffered.

Paraplegia: This refers to paralysis of the legs, usually due to a back injury severe enough to damage the lower spinal cord.

Quadriplegia: This is paralysis of all the extremities, usually as a result of spinal cord injury high in the neck. It is most often seen as a result of diving, cycling, and horse-riding injuries.

COMPLEMENTARY THERAPIES

Hydrotherapy

Every type of weakness and paralysis can be helped by some form of hydrotherapy. When inflammation is present, warm or hot baths will stimulate the circulation to the inflamed part. When there is nerve and muscle damage, swimming is effective in maximizing the use of the nerve and muscle units that succeeded in surviving the injury.

Acupressure

Stimulate large intestine 4 or 10, CV 6, lung 9, stomach 36, or kidney 3 for effective relief from symptoms.

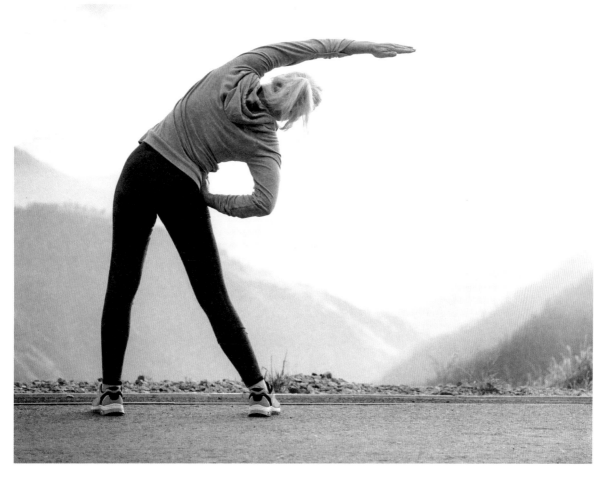

Exercise

Appropriate rest or restriction of activity is important when weakness is present, to avoid injury caused by a weakened muscle and to allow the body's healing mechanisms time to operate. After that time, gradual resumption of activity should be undertaken so that recovery is not unduly prolonged.

Yoga

Yoga has much to offer through its focus on the energy flow that arises from a union of body, mind, and spirit. Exercises that involve gentle stretching can firm and improve the functioning of muscles that have deteriorated following illness or injury.

Reflexology

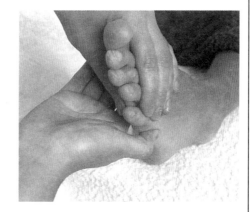

Careful movement of a paralyzed arm can be supplemented by thumb-walking the arm/leg reflex under the side of the little toe.

It is important that exercise be undertaken as soon as possible after injury so that the recovery period is not too prolonged.

LOSS OF CONSCIOUSNESS

There are a number of variations in the state of our consciousness, which we can define as the state of being awake and alert. Here we are talking about alterations in our ability to sense our immediate surroundings at any given moment in time.

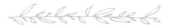

Conventional Therapies

- Anticonvulsant drugs
- Medical and surgical treatment of circulatory problems
- Surgical treatment of trauma and tumors
- Life-support measures

Let us look at some of the variations from the normal waking state.

"Absence" episodes: These are momentary lapses of consciousness, such as are seen in petit mal seizures; they barely interrupt the person's activities. No treatment of the episode is required, but the underlying situation needs to be understood and perhaps managed.

Fainting (syncope): There is a spectrum of symptoms here, ranging from feelings of faintness or giddiness to falling down in a "dead faint." The underlying causes are as follows: chemical, including hyperventilation and hypoglycemia; circulatory, stemming from either the heart or the peripheral blood vessels (this includes

First Aid

Keep the person in a recumbent position with any tight clothing loosened. Make sure that the airway is clear by observing the breathing, adjusting the position of the head, and removing mucus from the mouth. Open the windows to ensure adequate ventilation. If the person does not revive promptly, ready to resume normal activities, further measures may be necessary, including the use of emergency medical services.

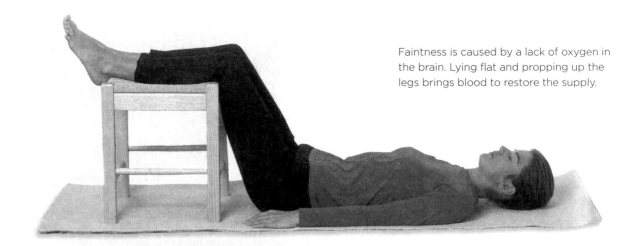

Faintness is caused by a lack of oxygen in the brain. Lying flat and propping up the legs brings blood to restore the supply.

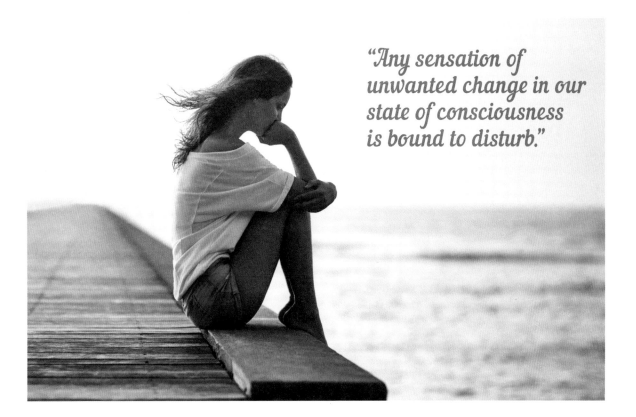

"Any sensation of unwanted change in our state of consciousness is bound to disturb."

the effects of emotional shock); and cerebral, including grand mal seizures and other causes.

Trance: A state between waking and sleeping, this term includes states induced by hypnosis and other conditions in which the "alpha state" is experienced, as in some meditative processes. Alpha state is that condition in which brain wave rhythms, measured at 13–30 cycles per second (cups) in the waking state, are slowed to 8–13 cups. Theta rhythm, measured at 4–7 cups, frequently appears in dreaming or in the half-waking hypnagogic state with dreamlike imagery. Delta rhythm, at ½–4 cups, is primarily associated with deep sleep.

Sleep: This is included for completeness only—it is of course normal and desirable. It differs from other states of lost consciousness in that a person can be roused from sleep, and once roused, can proceed with the usual range of waking-state activities.

Unconsciousness: This generally refers to a loss of consciousness from which the person cannot be roused for a period of time. It is most often seen in the setting of acute head injury or a vascular accident affecting the brain. It is self-limited and consciousness returns when the shock to the brain cells abates. Meanwhile, life-support systems may be required.

Coma: This is a state of unconsciousness that is profound and long-lasting. It is often accompanied by neurological signs of severe brain injury. Life-support measures must be used over a considerable period of time to sustain the patient's life.

SEE ALSO

Symptoms

- Chest pain page 56
- Circulatory symptoms page 98
- Seizures page 114
- Anxiety and panic page 130
- Phobias page 137
- Diabetic symptoms page 158
- Symptoms relating to immune function page 166

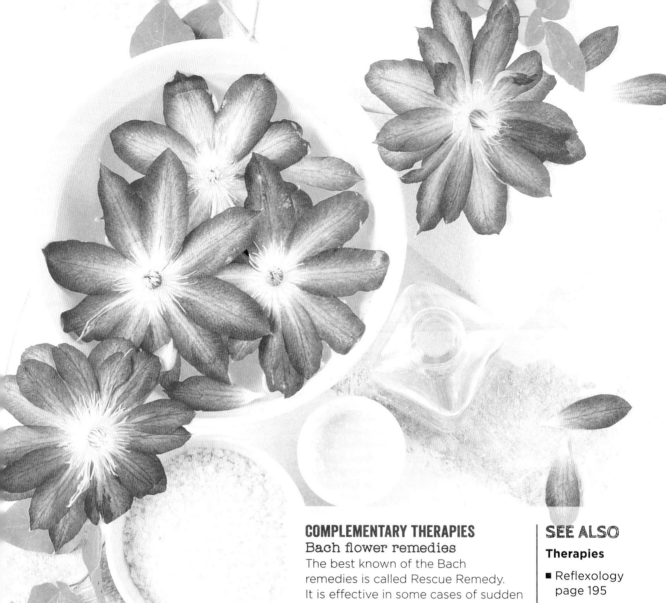

COMPLEMENTARY THERAPIES
Bach flower remedies

The best known of the Bach remedies is called Rescue Remedy. It is effective in some cases of sudden unconsciousness and is safe to use in all situations. Many people carry Rescue Remedy for use in this and similar emergencies. It is composed of the following:

- Cherry plum (fear of losing control)
- Clematis (to focus the mind and prevent fainting)
- Impatiens (impatience and tension)
- Rock rose (panic)
- Star of Bethlehem (shock)

Rescue Remedy is available in stock bottles with droppers from health food stores and herbal suppliers. Place four drops in the person's mouth, taking care not to touch his or her mouth with the dropper. You can repeat this every 10–15 minutes.

Bach Rescue Remedy is made from star of Bethlehem, clematis (above), cherry plum, rock rose, and impatiens.

SEE ALSO

Therapies

- Reflexology page 195

- Therapeutic touch page 212

- Imagery page 218

SLEEP-RELATED SYMPTOMS

The hours of sleep are the time for restoring all our bodily functions, or "recharging our batteries," on all levels of being—physical, mental, emotional, and spiritual. Sleep is one of the most natural functions in the cycle of life, yet millions of us seem to have great difficulty with it.

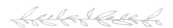

There are several conditions relating to sleep in which complementary therapies are helpful.

Insomnia: This is clearly the biggest problem of all. It divides into three categories: initial, interval, and terminal. Initial is when you are unable to get to sleep for a prolonged period. Almost invariably, this is connected with being unable to turn off the business of the day that is just concluding. All the worries, unresolved problems, and incomplete projects churn around in your head and sleep just will not come, seemingly for hours. Interval applies to awakening "in the middle of the night," and being unable to get back to sleep. Some people with this type get up, make a cup of cocoa, and then go back to bed. Terminal is when you wake up very early, still tired, but can get no more sleep. In some people, this is a sign of depression, especially if it occurs in association with other signs.

Sleep apnea: This is a rather unusual condition, seen almost always in overweight people. "Apnea" means "no breathing." In this condition the nose and throat seem to close up and prevent breathing for a number of seconds before the need for air practically forces the next breath.

This can be uncomfortable for the person and alarming for a partner. It seems to relate to excess fatty tissue in the neck region, but it is not completely understood.

Snoring: This is usually a problem for everybody but the snorer! It seems to be related to lying on the back while sleeping and to sleeping with the mouth open. Most snoring is produced by a fluttering of the soft palate. In children snoring may be associated with excess adenoidal tissue in the throat, producing habitual mouth-breathing.

Passionflower makes a good nightcap for restful sleep.

Conventional Therapies

- Sleep-inducing drugs
- Tranquilizers
- Over-the-counter sleeping preparations
- Treatment against infection, if present
- Attempts at weight control, if needed

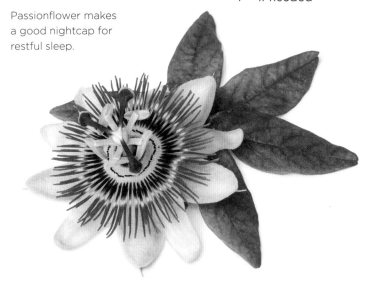

COMPLEMENTARY THERAPIES

Diet and nutrition

Melatonin is a natural substance produced by the pineal gland. In addition to its sleep benefits, it appears to have multiple other uses and minimal side-effects. Its safety is one of its most attractive characteristics. The suggestion has been made that the use of melatonin may affect the natural output of the pineal gland, the result of which is unclear. Therefore it may be best to restrict its use to people over 50 until further evidence is forthcoming. When it is taken in doses of 3–5mg within an hour of retiring, falling asleep is normalized and early awakening is improved or eliminated; there is no drowsiness or drugged feeling on awakening in the morning. It is available at health food stores and drugstores.

Weight control is an issue in sleep apnea. Many people with this problem are markedly overweight and have difficulty losing enough weight to make a difference to the symptom. A lifelong commitment to optimal nutrition and health is very worthwhile and tends to prevent problems such as this.

Meditation

The ability to seek and find inner calm is a significant factor in overcoming sleep problems for many people. The best way to approach this is not to wait until a problem arises, but rather to discover what method or methods suit you best and establish a daily practice.

Hydrotherapy

A soak in a hot bathtub within an hour of going to bed is a great way to relax and shed the cares of the day. Visualize all the thoughts and cares of the day rolling out of your pores into the water, leaving you clean inside and out!

Massage

The "cat stroke" is a calming massage to induce sleepiness.

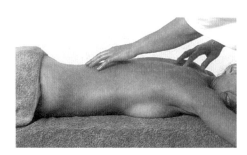

Start with both hands together, warming the sacrum reassuringly. Lightly slide one hand up the back and allow the other hand to follow on the other side.

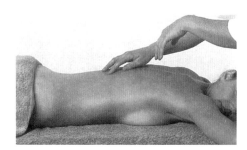

Slowly lift the hand that reaches the shoulders first, as the other hand continues to feather at a smooth pace up the back.

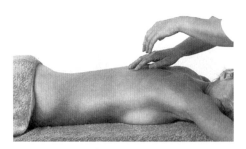

Allow the wrists to be loose and let each hand fall and rise gently from the relaxing body.

Aromatherapy

Add some oil of lavender, neroli, rose, or sweet marjoram to your bath, and relaxation will be even deeper. Alternatively, use these oils for self-massage of the face, neck, and shoulders. Finish up with a few drops of lavender or neroli oil on your pillow.

Herbal therapy

Lemon balm, chamomile, lime blossom, and/or passionflower are excellent when drunk as tea before sliding into bed.

Exercise

Maintaining an active, healthy life is a strong promoter of good sleep patterns by a variety of means.

- It promotes oxygenation of all tissues.
- It keeps muscles in tone and joints limber.
- It imparts a sense of well-being.
- It helps to balance food intake and normalize body weight.

Choose the kinds of exercise that suit you best and partake every day!

"*Sleep is the great natural restorer of our physical and mental well-being.*"

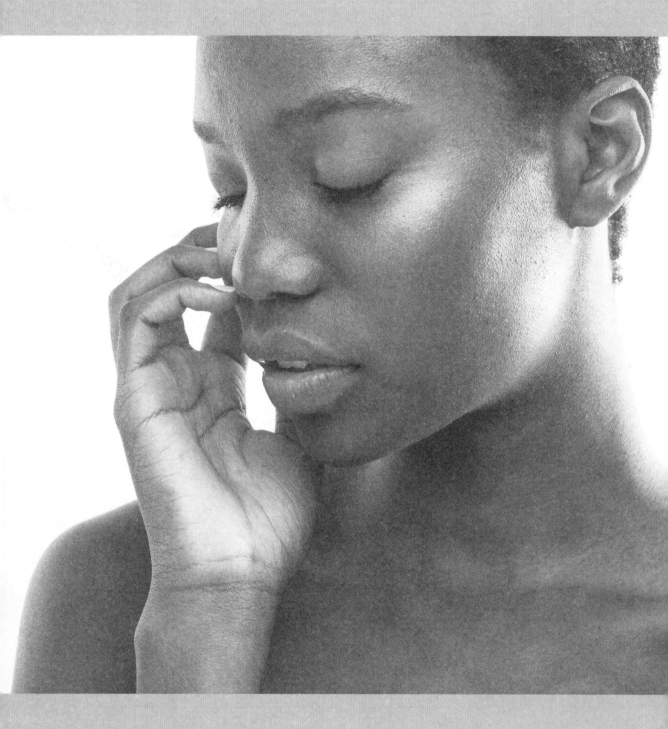

EMOTIONAL & SPIRITUAL

ANXIETY AND PANIC

Anxiety, in all its forms and disguises, is certainly the dominant symptom of our era. The drugs prescribed to control or suppress it have been bestsellers for decades. Only in the past few years has a significant amount of research gone into the reasons behind this condition and its unremitting rise.

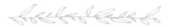

Conventional Therapies

- Psychotropic drugs
- Counseling and psychotherapy
- Removal of the person from the inciting atmosphere to more neutral surroundings

Two statements, flowing partly from this research, can be made with reasonable accuracy.
- The causes of anxiety are far too numerous to list and in any particular case are specific to its circumstances and history. You know if you are suffering from anxiety and your case is not a carbon copy of anybody else's—it is unique.

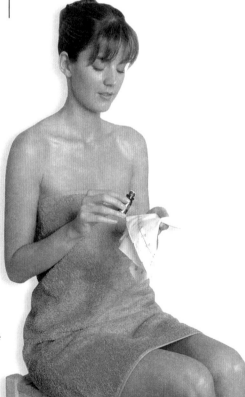

Inhaling a suitable essential oil from a handkerchief can help calm some of the symptoms of anxiety.

- Anxiety can be eliminated from our experience without toxic drugs. It is a premise of this book that even in the direst of circumstances, anxiety only complicates matters and is really an unnecessary and unwanted response to trials and tribulations. These will not go away, but there are better ways of coping with them.

One generalization about anxiety seems justified—behind all its manifestations lies an element of fear that we may or may not recognize, or may even deny. Identifying the fear and its roots may lead to acceptance of it and allow the sufferer to feel more at ease.

Let us look at some of the varieties and gradations of anxiety that people experience, in general categories.

Nervousness: This rather mild form of anxiety can be connected with a lot of other feelings that are familiar to all of us, including shyness, lack of confidence, insecurity, feelings of inadequacy, and social clumsiness. These may progress to more serious problems or may recede into the background as we grow.

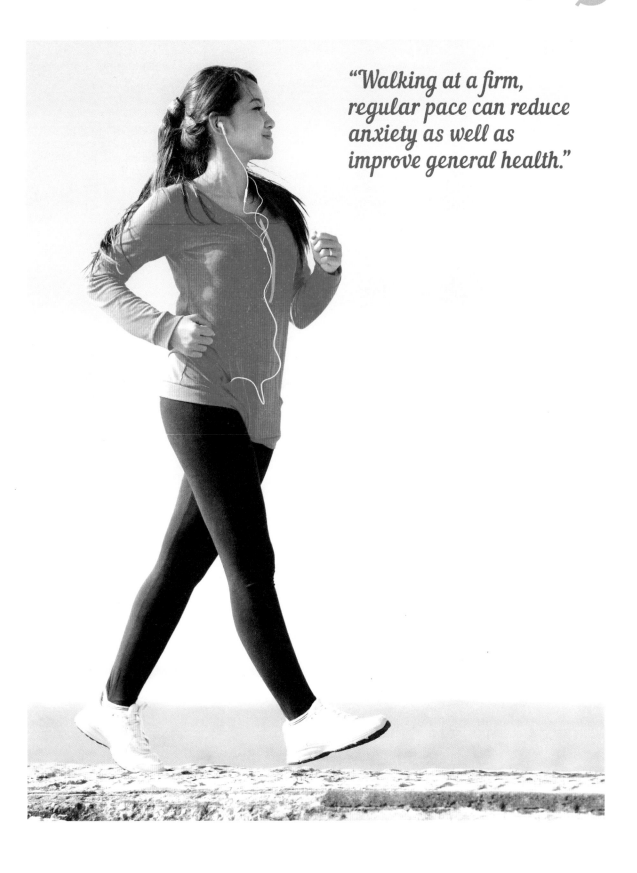

"Walking at a firm, regular pace can reduce anxiety as well as improve general health."

Lavender is renowned for its calming effects, and can be used in massage oils, for inhalations, and also in baths.

Genuine anxiety: This is when people begin to feel threatened and out of control because of their feelings about themselves and their surroundings. There is a low-level background of discomfort that they cannot seem to shake off. It may go on for months or years, never reaching crisis proportions but never going away. It is possible to live like this, but it causes wear and tear on the emotional system and leads to impaired peformance in the workplace and in relationships. It is reversible, but often the sufferer does not know that.

Panic: This is a more extreme and acute version that fortunately most people do not have to endure. It is very much like the panic of being trapped in a burning building. The anxious feelings start to accumulate when the sufferer has lost some of the energy formerly used to cope with them. The person eventually feels surrounded and unable to escape as he or she could before. An unpleasant panic reaction follows, replete with physical symptoms of discomfort: racing heart, rapid breathing, excessive sweating, clouded thinking—to name but a few. Even this extreme situation can be managed, but it often takes the help of others to find the way out.

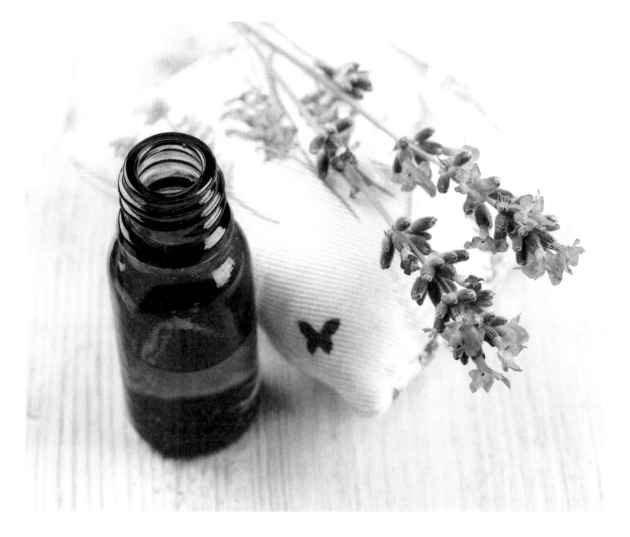

COMPLEMENTARY THERAPIES

Aromatherapy

Add any of the following to your bath to experience a calming effect: ylang-ylang, geranium, rose, neroli, melissa, lavender, sandalwood, or patchouli. You can also use these oils in conjunction with a relaxing body massage or inhale them from a tissue or your pillow.

Exercise

Walking at a heart rate of 100 beats per minute is effective in reducing levels of anxiety. This is a happy circumstance as it works in many ways to promote optimal health. Exercise at whatever level lowers the level of the bodily symptoms you may experience with anxiety.

Diet and nutrition

- The consistent following of an optimal nutritional program is effective in the prevention of anxiety and the maintenance of mental and emotional balance. Avoiding caffeine reduces anxiety.
- The amino acid acetyl L-carnitine is safe and effective against neuropsychiatric symptoms in doses of 250mg one to four times daily. It is available in health food stores.

Meditation

Many studies have shown the positive value of meditation in preserving a state of mental and emotional balance and in relieving the symptoms of emotional distress. It is best to establish which of the many methods suits you best when you are feeling well, and then to practice that method daily. At times of increased anxiety, your meditative technique will be there to call upon.

Massage

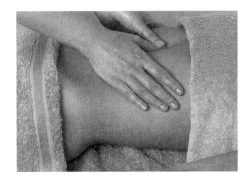

The solar plexus (the soft triangular hollow under the ribs) can be tender at times of stress. Gently circle the thumbs there, one on top of the other, with fingers on the outer rib cage.

Biofeedback

Biofeedback training is demonstrably effective in controlling symptoms of anxiety. It is a proven technique with many years of experience behind it. You will need a qualified trainer to start you off and a small amount of equipment. Then you will be able to use the technique on your own at home.

Hydrotherapy

Warm and hot soaking baths have been known for generations for their soothing, anti-anxiety properties. They work in various ways.

- They relax tight muscles and slow the racing heart.
- They separate you from the turbulent atmosphere in which you were struggling.
- They lead you toward a sense of well-being and provide time for your inner healing mechanisms to operate.

DEPRESSION

Depression is a widespread problem in our society, extending from feelings of being somewhat tired and "blue" to a major psychiatric illness lasting months to years. In its milder form, depression can be seen as merely an exaggeration of the mood swings that we all feel during the ebb and flow of everyday events. We recover after a healthy meal and a good night's sleep.

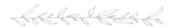

Conventional Therapies

- Antidepressant drugs
- Counseling and psychotherapy
- Removal from the inciting atmosphere (e.g. to hospital)
- Extreme measures, such as shock therapy

The person who has a more serious problem does not become better with these simple measures. Life's problems look even bigger and depression deepens. Concentration is lost, irritability enters the picture, and judgment is affected. Loss of appetite, constipation, and insomnia appear. Finally, the person feels completely helpless and without hope.

At any point in this descent, depression may start to turn around of its own accord, taking on the appearance of a cyclical affair. It may be an aspect of bipolar illness, which is cyclical in nature. In any case, it does appear that the body's gyroscope, the part that keeps things on an even keel, has lost some of its power to steady. In reality, our whole being is that gyroscope and we need to use every means available to restore strength, integrity, and balance. In short, we must strive to restore optimal health.

"Depression can strike in mild or severe form and requires treatment of the whole body."

COMPLEMENTARY THERAPIES

Diet and nutrition

An optimal nutrition program is highly desirable for the prevention and management of depression, because it helps to keep mood swings within a balanced range. Reduced levels of the following have been found in some people with depression: magnesium, phenylalanine, vitamin B2, vitamin B6, vitamin B12, folic acid, and thyroid hormone. Many classes of drugs can reduce vitamin levels in the body, paving the way for depression, among them the very drugs used to treat depression.

Biofeedback

Biofeedback training is effective in managing the symptoms of depression. You need a qualified trainer initially and must buy a small amount of equipment. You can then use the method at home whenever you need it.

Meditation

The ability to go to the calm quiet place within you is a valuable asset in depression. Learn how to do this when you are feeling well so that you can access it easily when you feel down.

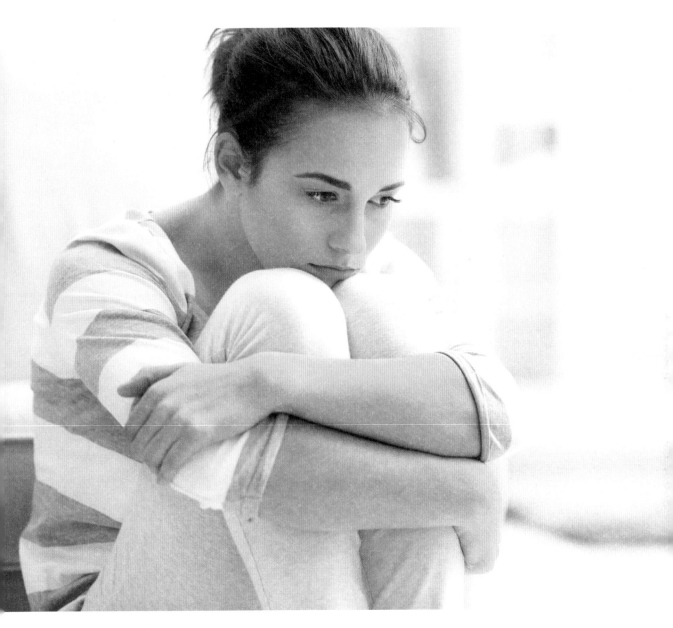

Stress management

It is important to consider lifestyle issues, such as interpersonal relationships at home and in the workplace, when trying to resolve depression. Keep in mind that it is easier to evaluate your situation in a balanced way and to resolve any conflicts that exist when you are feeling well rather than when you are not.

Exercise

Exercise has been shown to lighten depression. The most accessible form of exercise for everyone is walking, though you may have another particular favorite. You will get the most consistent results by selecting the level of exercise that is right for you and practicing it every day.

Mental and emotional pain can be as painful as physical pain—and often far harder to bear, especially if you are alone.

Reflexology

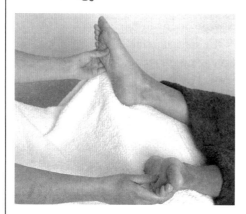

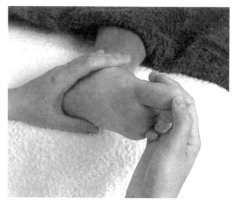

Let your thumbs fall into each foot's solar plexus point, under and between the second and third toes. Push toward the person on an in-breath, and let the feet flop on an out-breath.

Thumb-walk all over the "head " of each toe, especially the first (big) toe, to relax a tired or aching brain. The area may be hard in the depressed, who are too centered on the head.

Aromatherapy

The following can be used in massage oils or in the bathtub to lift the spirits: jasmine, clary sage, ylang-ylang, bergamot, neroli, rose, orange, lemon, and lavender.

Herbal therapy

- Basil
- Borage
- Lemon balm
- Lime blossom
- Skullcap
- St. John's wort (*Hypericum*)

Bach flower remedies

These remedies can be taken from the stock bottle or diluted in water, by themselves or in combination.
- Gorse (hopelessness)
- Sweet chestnut (deep despair)
- Willow (bitter resentment)

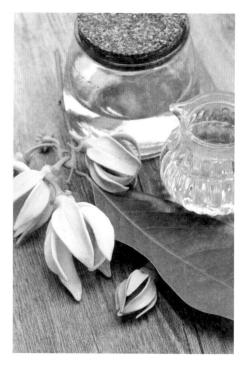

Ylang-ylang is known to lift the spirits and can be useful in the alleviation of the symptoms of depression.

PHOBIAS

Fear is said by many to be at the root of much of the unease people feel, especially in a fast-moving, confusing, and complex society such as ours. At the surface are specific fears we are very much aware of, such as fear of snakes, spiders, heights, and crowds. At deeper levels, there are said to be more formless fears of which the superficial ones may be but symbols—fear of illness, failure, and death itself.

These things are probably present in all of us, but some people are clearly more affected by them than others. Perhaps a trauma has pushed some of the deeper feelings to the surface, where they create much disturbance in our equilibrium. Those who suffer with phobias can be severely disabled by them. They sometimes surface as panic attacks, when the underlying fear produces a sharp buzz of anxiety that can be nearly overwhelming.

COMPLEMENTARY THERAPIES

Diet and nutrition

Specific attention has been drawn to the possibility of hypoglycemia. It may be useful to test this by strictly avoiding foods containing sugar and white flour for a long enough period to determine whether there is a connection.

Imagery

This involves learning to visualize yourself doing the thing that you fear. It must be learned with the help of an experienced person. Once the imagery is securely in place, it can be reinforced indefinitely at home on one's own.

Group therapy

Various groups exist to help phobia sufferers, both to offer specific therapy programs and to bring people together for mutual support. An important part of some groups is putting the affected person through a "desensitization" program. This involves leading the person through the experience that the person fears. This is done gradually and gently until the person can tolerate the experience for longer periods, accompanied by fewer people and finally alone. This is not a panacea, but it does help some people.

Meditation

It is important for a phobia sufferer to experience inner strength and integration. A regular practice of "going within" is sure to bring one into that valuable dimension, the quiet, calm center of being.

Conventional Therapies

- Tranquilizers and sedatives
- Counseling and psychotherapy

SEE ALSO

Symptoms

- Sleep-related symptoms page 125
- Anxiety and panic page 130

Therapies

- Yoga page 204
- Stress management page 220
- Bach flower remedies page 236

ADDICTIONS

The subject of addictions is wide-ranging. It embraces the world of drug use and abuse and also the vast realms of personality and human interactions. The term implies dependency, but more than that, it specifically connotes the basic element of appetite.

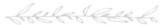

Conventional Therapies

- Tranquilizers and antidepressant drugs

- 12-step programs, of which the prototype is Alcoholics Anonymous

- Support groups

If a person is addicted, whether to food, drugs, or to a self-defeating attitude or relationship, that person feels an increasing need for the object of his or her addiction and suffers prolonged physical and emotional torment when that object is withheld. In the latter situation, the person is said to suffer withdrawal symptoms. This strongly suggests the involvement of many of the body's internal systems in what appeared initially to stem from the realm of thoughts and desires.

One message that is beamed at us from our materialistic culture is that there are many "things" we need to make our lives complete. This appeals to the part of us that would like to blame what is wrong in our lives on something external, or the lack of it. The intent of this message is to addict us to the things of the material world. The core of addiction is the idea that there are hollow places within us that are labeled "Aching Need," and that various items can be poured in to fill up the holes and take the ache away. There are many items that we see people reach out for to fill their "needs."

- **Food:** This is usually an attempt to assuage loneliness and depression.
- **Drugs and alcohol:** These are to dull the awareness of how bad things are.
- **Objects:** These impart feelings of power and are showy extensions of themselves.
- **People:** These are to make them feel accepted and supported in their weakness and inadequacy.

Another idea that the culture conveys is that "more is better." So when people pour these things into the holes they perceive inside themselves, they may feel better for a while, but then the old, empty, aching feelings return. Because "more is better," they conclude that they just need to put more of the same into the hole the next time, and so the process goes on.

The truth of the matter is that we already have within us the potential to be complete. The power we need is in here, not out there! The only tool we need to access that power is the knowlege and belief that we have it.

COMPLEMENTARY THERAPIES
Group therapy

Many people find that meeting with others who are similarly challenged is very helpful, as it provides a forum of ideas and forges a community around common issues. Many communities have printed or electronic bulletin boards that provide the necessary information.

"Smoking is one of the most common addictions—and one of the hardest to break."

Stress management

It is useful to take a frank look at how we relate to the significant people in our lives and also at our life in the workplace, because these people and situations are likely to be associated with most of our stress. Ask yourself if you are engaging in relationships in the fairest and most loving ways, and whether your work gives you a real sense of vocation and affirmation. The answers to these questions will go a long way toward strengthening your connections with others in a way that preserves integrity and dignity for you and them.

Exercise

It is important in terms of a sense of well-being to establish an appropriate exercise program and to engage in it on a daily basis. This also plays a significant part alongside nutrition in the preservation of ideal body weight.

Diet and nutrition

An optimal nutrition program is one of the cornerstones of good health, giving energy and stamina for the tasks we are called upon to perform. A sense of strength and adequacy is a fundamental part of appreciating our wholeness and resisting the notion that we have missing pieces that can be supplied from outside.

A secondary issue, but one of significance to many, is the maintenance of body weight within reasonable limits. In this context the benefits in terms of self-image and self-confidence go beyond the undeniable health benefits.

Aromatherapy

Used in an early morning bath, a few drops of any of the following essential oils will stimulate energy release and give you a boost: basil, rosemary, clary sage, and peppermint.

Bach flower remedies

Larch will help you to stiffen your resolve when trying to quit an addiction.

Herbal therapy

The following herbs support the nervous system when we feel exhausted and most susceptible to the addictive process.
- Drink infusions of oats, vervain, licorice, or skullcap three times a day, while avoiding caffeine, alcohol, and tobacco, to help support the nervous system and exhausted adrenal glands.
- Dandelion, burdock, and red clover will cleanse the system, especially after too much caffeine or alcohol.
- Ginseng and astragalus boost physical energy in the face of fatigue and nervous exhaustion.

Astragalus, combined with ginseng, helps to boost physical energy and is a good alternative to caffeine or alcohol.

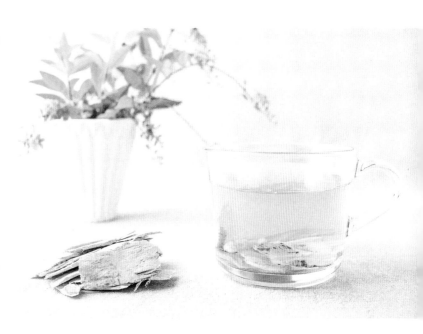

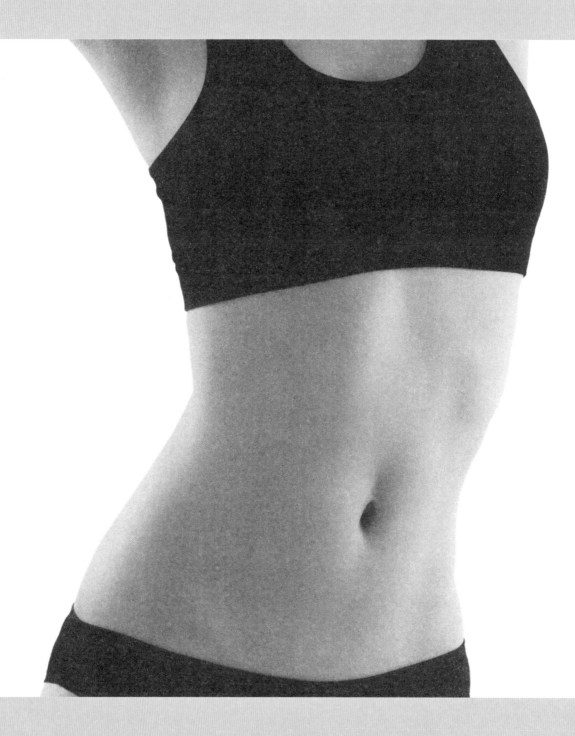

DIGESTIVE SYSTEM

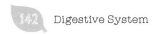

EATING DISORDERS

Apart from considerations of the content of a diet and nutrition program, there are a few conditions concerning people's attitudes to food and their eating habits. These produce marked variations in the intake of food, thus affecting health in a different way from the subtle metabolic changes that are discussed under Diet and Nutrition (page 175).

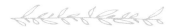

Conventional Therapies

- Psychotropic drugs and sedatives

- Psychotherapy and psychiatry

- Medical therapy of any underlying illness

Below are some of the symptoms that relate to variations in the intake of food and drink.

Excessive appetite: This is associated with overactivity of the thyroid, some instances of diabetes mellitus, and compulsive overeating. (The issue of excess weight is covered elsewhere.)

Reduced appetite: This occurs in many situations. The vast majority of acute illnesses are characterized by some loss of appetite. It is a serious symptom in a few, such as cancer and depression, where it may be prolonged and materially affect the outcome.

Anorexia nervosa: This disorder has received considerable attention in the past few years. It is increasingly seen as a symptom of the interaction of people (principally women) with their culture, which erects artificial standards that people strive to meet to an extent that is detrimental to health. This disorder involves voluntary restriction of food intake, which sometimes reaches the point of starvation.

Bulimia: This is a variation of the anorexia theme, in which food intake may be more or less normal but induced vomiting is regularly practiced, producing a similar effect. Both of these conditions reflect a person enduring a marked degree of stress. These conditions indicate a life seriously out of balance.

Extreme diet variations: There are a number of ways in which people, for various reasons, adopt dietary programs that are quite deficient in essential nutrients. The reasons for the use of these variations, whether singly or in combination, include the following.

- Illness may necessitate the use of such a diet—for example, a macrobiotic diet for cancer. In this instance, short-term use may have detoxifying properties, while long-term use could be challenged as nutritionally unsound.

- Fasting can be detoxifying in the short run, depleting in the long run.

- Ignorance is another category. The innocent (and perhaps unsupervised) teenager who seems unaware that a diet of french fries and colas is very unhealthy could be put here.

"Counseling and group therapy are used to explore the basis of eating disorders, which often arise from difficulties in personal relationships."

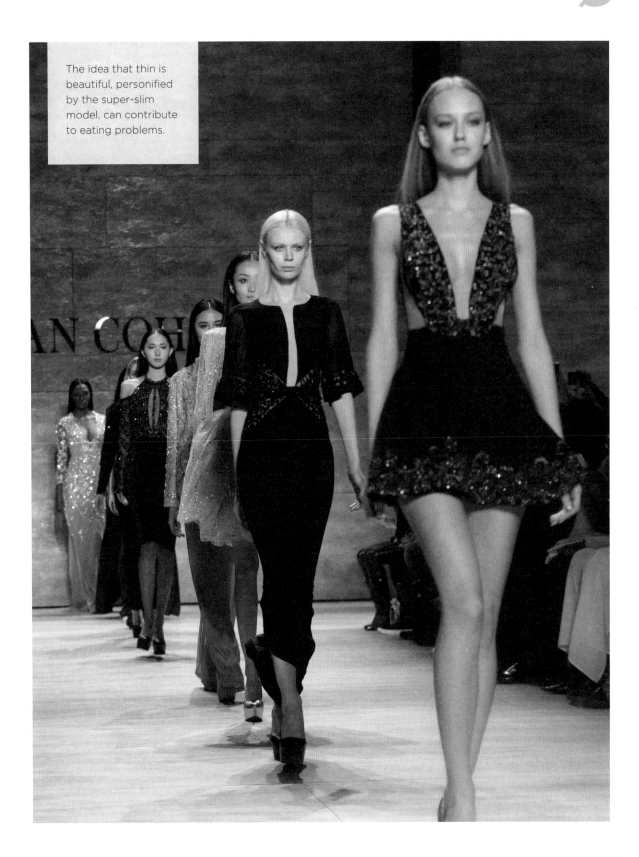

The idea that thin is beautiful, personified by the super-slim model, can contribute to eating problems.

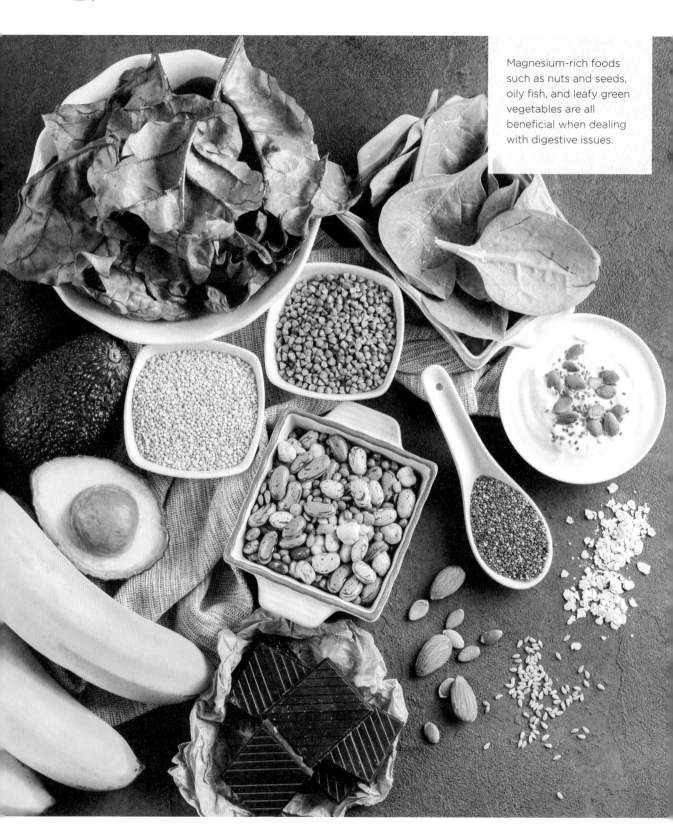

Magnesium-rich foods such as nuts and seeds, oily fish, and leafy green vegetables are all beneficial when dealing with digestive issues.

COMPLEMENTARY THERAPIES
Group therapy
Anorexia nervosa and bulimia should improve in the context of group therapy, where the support of others similarly afflicted is a key feature.

Diet and nutrition
While it is obvious that an optimal nutrition program is needed here, a few specifics can be mentioned.

- Magnesium deficiency can be produced by anorexia or bulimia, with resulting weakness, nausea, depression, and other symptoms. Adequate supplementation can prevent these.
- Zinc deficiency appears to exist in anorexia nervosa; supplementation at 45mg per day has been shown to result in significant weight gain.
- Vitamin B12 deficiency can be a cause as well as a symptom of anorexia.

Exercise
A program of appropriate exercise is effective in stimulating appetite, combating depression, and promoting ideal weight. Brisk walking and swimming are ideal for all but those who are bedridden.

Meditation
The ability to seek and find the serene center of one's being through daily practice is desirable in all circumstances, and these conditions are no exception. The inner self contains the proper healthy image of the person, so it is important to be able to connect with that image repeatedly on a daily basis.

Stress management
Difficulties in relationships at home or in the workplace are often at the root of serious eating disturbances. It is as well to look thoroughly at these personal interactions, since the symptom may be a signpost pointing the way to positive changes and better things ahead.

Herbal therapy
- Astragalus stimulates appetite.
- Goldenseal is useful for loss of appetite, but should be avoided during pregnancy.
- St. John's wort (*Hypericum*) brings improvement in anorexia.
- Mix equal parts of juniper berries, balm leaves, European centaury, and nettle leaves and steep 1 teaspoon in $\frac{1}{2}$ cup boiling water. Take $\frac{1}{2}$–1 cup a day, sweetened with honey, in mouthful doses to help stimulate appetite.

SEE ALSO
Symptoms

- Anxiety and panic page 130
- Depression page 134
- Addictions page 138
- Weight disorders page 146
- Diabetic symptoms page 158

Therapies

- Anxiety and panic page 130
- Depression page 134
- Addictions page 138
- Weight disorders page 146
- Diabetic symptoms page 158

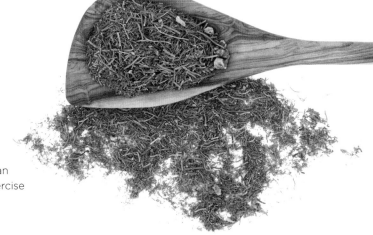

The herb goldenseal is often used for treating loss of appetite and can be combined with appropriate exercise for even better results.

WEIGHT DISORDERS

Body weight has been a preoccupation in our culture for quite a long time. Obesity is clearly implicated as an aggravating factor in a number of our most common unhealthy conditions, and being underweight is now increasingly encountered as an inciting cause of illness, especially among people who are very aggressive in areas of fitness.

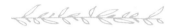

Conventional Therapies

- Appetite-suppressing drugs
- Low-calorie diets
- Exercise
- Fitness clinics
- Surgery in extreme cases

Hundreds of books and thousands of articles have each proposed a slightly different way to control weight. A few simple statements will give an overview of this quite complex subject.

- Eating too much food, and the wrong kind of food, leads to an unhealthy weight and then to obesity, which has distinct health ramifications, such as diabetes and hypertension.
- Weight has a particular relationship to diabetes that creates an unhealthy cycle. Obesity is characterized by resistance to the effects of insulin, leading to impaired glucose tolerance (a feature of diabetes) and diminished eating-related heat generation. This leads to further weight gain, and so on.
- Being overweight is the greatest single lifestyle factor associated with high blood pressure: 20–30 percent of hypertension is attributable to excess weight.

- Exercise levels are directly linked to food intake levels in the maintenance of a healthy body weight range. Different forms of exercise vary in their ability to control weight.
- Undereating and overtraining, while not as hazardous to health as their opposites, can produce their own set of health consequences, such as dietary deficiency and loss of menses.

As in all things, finding the right balance in the management of body weight is the key to a healthy state. Clearly those at the extremes of the weight range are the least healthy.

At the same time, it must also be said that a person should maintain his or her weight at a level that gives psychological comfort, i.e. where body mass best conforms to body image. This point can be very hard to define and is subject to many outside influences that are not necessarily health-inducing. Many people, for example, are thrown into turmoil when they compare clothing ads with the image they see in the mirror.

Another important aspect is that one person may be quite fit, on the basis of an optimal nutrition program and an appropriate exercise program, while another person of the same

"Loss of weight has consistently been found to bring about a reduction in blood pressure."

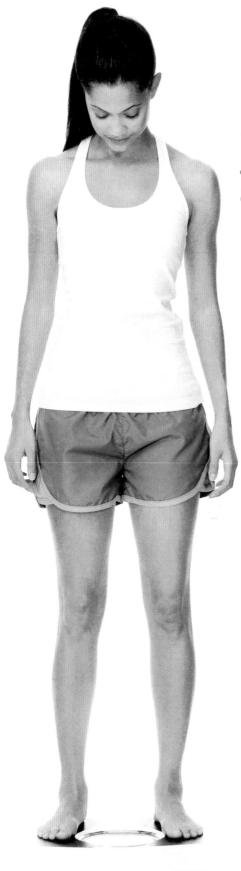

"The needle on the weighing scale is a useful indicator but not the only clue to healthy weight."

height and weight may have very unhealthy arteries and internal organs due to poor diet, and be badly out of condition due to lack of an exercise program. The latter person may be easy to spot, having poor posture, a protuberant abdomen, sallow, oily skin, and possibly slight wheezing. So it is not simply a matter of how far the needle moves on the weighing scale that determines health, although it can be one helpful indicator of our overall state of health and fitness.

COMPLEMENTARY THERAPIES
Diet and nutrition

In conjunction with a healthy diet program, a few specific points of interest can be noted.

- L-carnitine and chromium picolinate have brought about weight reduction in studies where the calorie intake is held constant.
- Users of artificial sweeteners were found in a large study to be more likely than non-users to gain weight. Contrary to what might have been expected, the differences were not attributable to food consumption patterns and no other explanation was postulated. One can only speculate about the cause of this finding.
- The substance known as 5-hydroxy tryptophan has been used successfully in weight reduction, but its use is controversial.

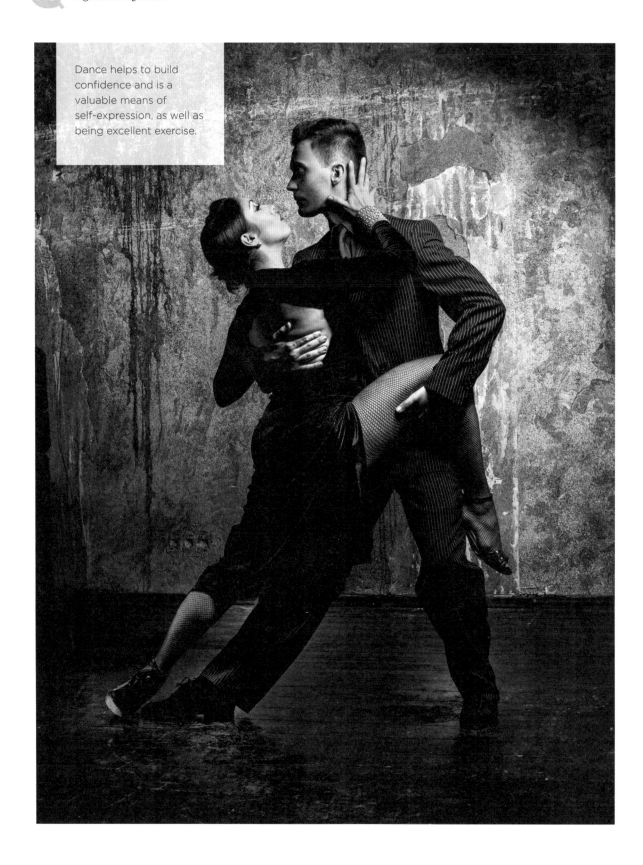

Dance helps to build confidence and is a valuable means of self-expression, as well as being excellent exercise.

Exercise

- Calorie restriction plus brisk exercise results in loss of fat only, while dieting alone results in loss of muscle mass as well as fat, leading to deconditioning.
- Brisk walking and cycling lead to greater weight loss than the exercise of swimming laps.
- Dance can provide exercise while also being a valuable means of self-expression.
- Use your exercise for pleasure and not to strive after perfection.

Meditation

The ability to seek and find the calmness at the center of one's being is important to the restoration of healthy balances in the body, including that involved in body weight. Discover which method suits you best, then establish a regular practice.

Imagery

Imagery has been found to be very effective in altering unhealthy habit patterns such as overeating. The technique must be properly learned, after which you can practice it on your own, whenever you like, and for as long a period of time as necessary.

Herbal therapy

Guggul derivatives have brought about weight loss.

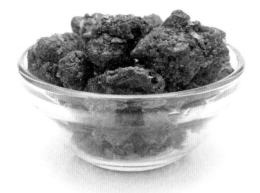

Acupressure

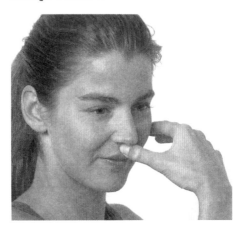

Press the center of the groove between nose and lip for 7–10 seconds to encourage weight loss while following a healthy diet program.

Massage

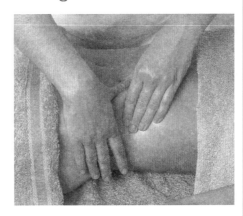

Knead fleshier areas, such as buttocks, thighs, knees, and sides of the abdomen, to help tone muscles and maximize fat loss from good exercise.

The guggul plant is most common in northern India. It can be used to aid weight loss.

SEE ALSO

Symptoms

- Blood pressure page 59
- Anxiety and panic page 130
- Addictions page 138
- Eating disorders page 142
- Diabetic symptoms page 158

Therapies

- Alexander technique page 185
- Yoga page 204
- Stress management page 220
- Group therapy page 223

NAUSEA AND VOMITING

Nausea and vomiting, while they can occur separately, are so closely allied that for practical purposes they can be considered as one symptom. They constitute an early indication that something is going amiss internally, hence their importance. Vomiting is usually, but not always, preceded by nausea.

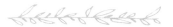

Conventional Therapies

- Antispasmodic and sedative drugs
- Medical treatment of any underlying illness

SEE ALSO

Symptoms

- Infections page 50
- Abdominal pain page 78
- Anxiety and panic page 130
- Eating disorders page 142

Therapies

- Diet and nutrition page 175
- Bach flower remedies page 236

Nausea may be associated with pallor of the skin, increased perspiration and salivation, and sometimes lowering of blood pressure and slowing of the heart. Vomiting results from the stimulation of the one or more centers in the brain that control the structures involved in the act of vomiting. Thus a number of varied conditions can activate the vomiting centers.

A variety of conditions can produce nausea and vomiting, as follows:

- Acute infections, e.g. flu, ear infections, and gastroenteritis
- Acute conditions in the abdomen, e.g. appendicitis, gallstone, kidney stone, and ulcer
- Congestive heart failure due to congestion of abdominal organs
- Metabolic conditions, e.g. pregnancy, diabetes, and uremia
- Nervous system disorders, e.g. meningitis, labyrinthitis, and migraine
- Numerous drugs and poisons
- Emotional disturbances, e.g. nervous upsets and anorexia/bulimia

COMPLEMENTARY THERAPIES
Meditation

Acute illness, which is so often the setting for nausea and vomiting, is in itself a significant stress factor. If one can connect with the calm center of one's being when illness strikes, the severity of the attack is lessened. It is best to discover the method that suits you when you are well and to practice daily, so that the pathway is open and ready to access when it is needed.

Reflexology

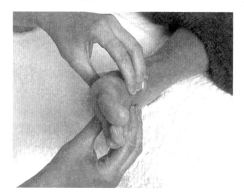

To treat nausea, support the foot underneath with the thumbs and finger-walk all the fingers out from the center top of the foot, working from ankle tip to toes. Next, finger-walk in lines between each toe before gently pinching that area.

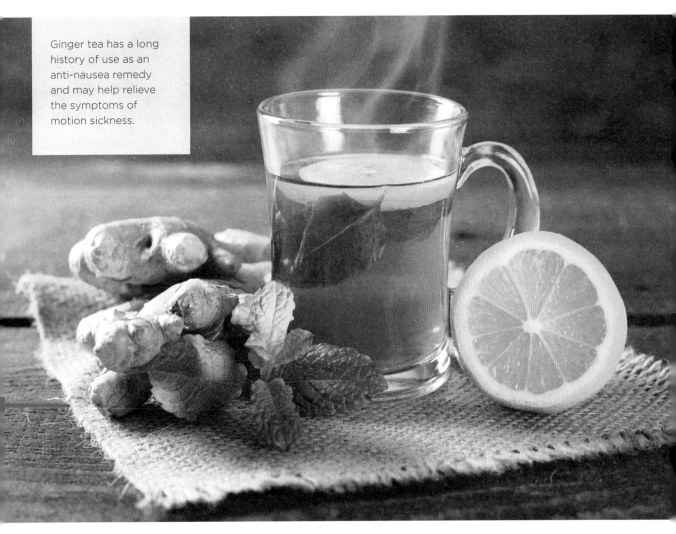

Ginger tea has a long history of use as an anti-nausea remedy and may help relieve the symptoms of motion sickness.

Homeopathy

This combination has been found effective in vertigo with nausea.

- Cocculus D4—210mg
- Ambra D6—30mg
- Conuma D3—30mg
- Mineral oil D8—30mg

Herbal therapy

- Feverfew (migraine)
- Ginger (motion sickness)

Acupressure

The acupressure wristband is effective in motion sickness and pernicious vomiting.

"The acupressure wristband can successfully combat certain forms of nausea."

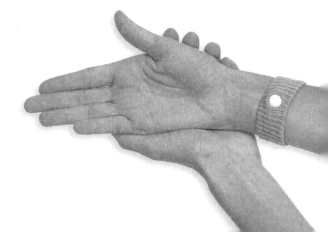

INDIGESTION

If one can judge from media advertising, indigestion must be one of the most prevalent disorders in our culture today. As the term implies, it relates to the difficulties the body has in processing what has entered the mouth, be it food, drink, or drug. It is a rather imprecise term, since it is so subjective and related to the individual's experience.

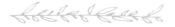

Conventional Therapies

- Drugs that either block the production of gastric acid or neutralize it
- Drugs against spasm and/or gas
- Restricted diets
- Surgery

Most people experience indigestion as one of the following symptoms.

Heartburn: This is a hot sensation at the lower end of the breastbone or extending up into the chest for several inches. It may be accompanied by acid regurgitation into the back of the throat and is sometimes called acid indigestion.

Stomachache: This is more of a crampy feeling in the upper abdomen after certain foods. It is often related to excesses of coffee or tea, but it can follow other foods. An upper abdominal pain on an empty stomach is more likely to reflect inflammation at the outlet of the stomach into the duodenum, the place where most ulcers occur.

Bloated feeling: A frequent comment is: "I feel as though I was blown up with a bicycle pump." In most cases, the feeling is caused by excess gas, a by-product of incomplete digestion. There may be excessive gurgling as well.

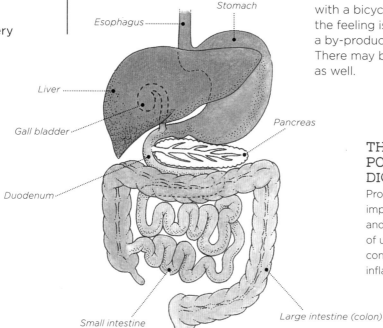

Esophagus

Stomach

Liver

Gall bladder

Pancreas

Duodenum

Small intestine

Large intestine (colon)

Rectum

THE ABDOMINAL PORTION OF THE DIGESTIVE TRACT

Problems here are often imprecisely labeled "indigestion," and can range from the results of unwise or over-hasty food consumpion to stress-related inflammation and ulcers.

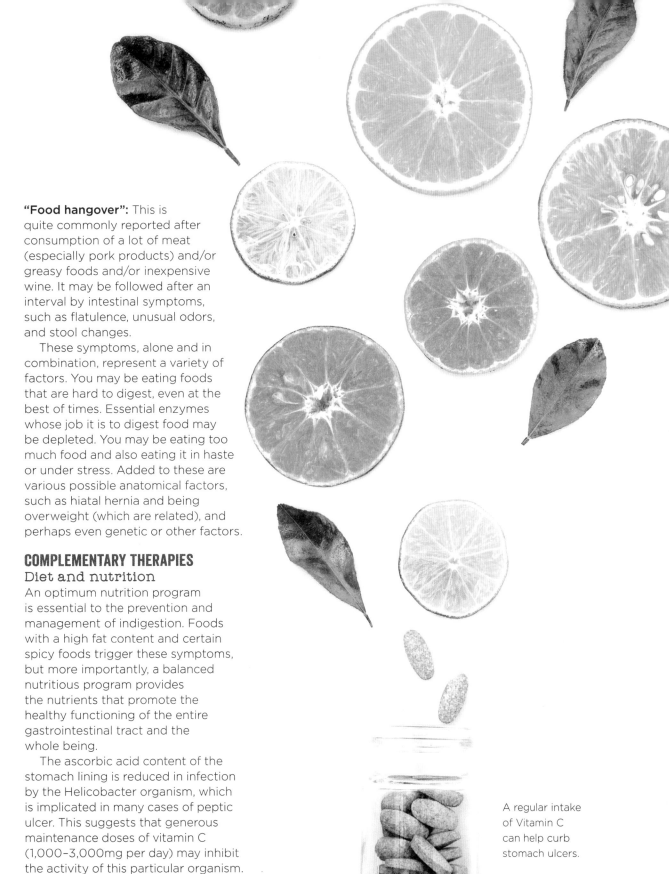

"Food hangover": This is quite commonly reported after consumption of a lot of meat (especially pork products) and/or greasy foods and/or inexpensive wine. It may be followed after an interval by intestinal symptoms, such as flatulence, unusual odors, and stool changes.

These symptoms, alone and in combination, represent a variety of factors. You may be eating foods that are hard to digest, even at the best of times. Essential enzymes whose job it is to digest food may be depleted. You may be eating too much food and also eating it in haste or under stress. Added to these are various possible anatomical factors, such as hiatal hernia and being overweight (which are related), and perhaps even genetic or other factors.

COMPLEMENTARY THERAPIES
Diet and nutrition
An optimum nutrition program is essential to the prevention and management of indigestion. Foods with a high fat content and certain spicy foods trigger these symptoms, but more importantly, a balanced nutritious program provides the nutrients that promote the healthy functioning of the entire gastrointestinal tract and the whole being.

The ascorbic acid content of the stomach lining is reduced in infection by the Helicobacter organism, which is implicated in many cases of peptic ulcer. This suggests that generous maintenance doses of vitamin C (1,000–3,000mg per day) may inhibit the activity of this particular organism.

A regular intake of Vitamin C can help curb stomach ulcers.

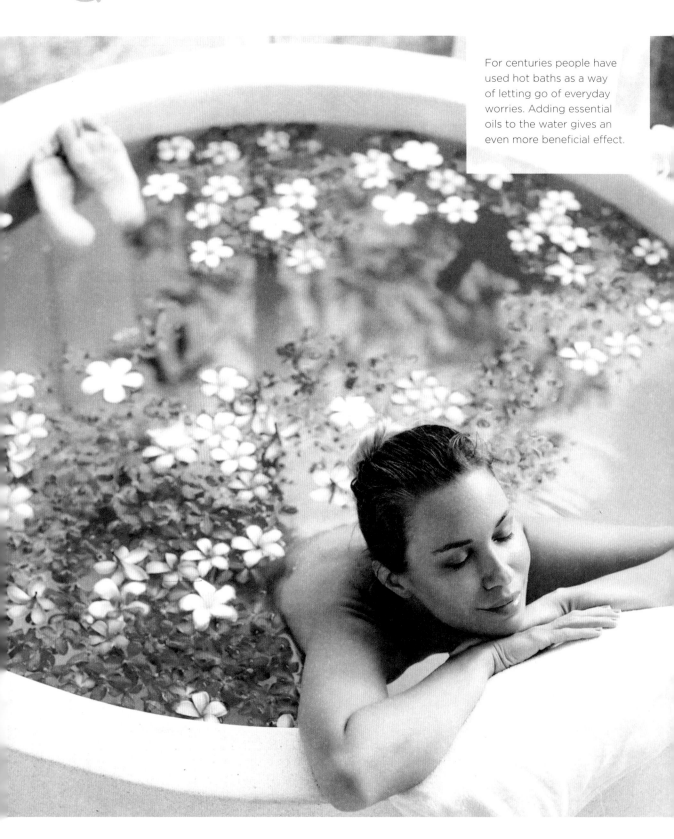

For centuries people have used hot baths as a way of letting go of everyday worries. Adding essential oils to the water gives an even more beneficial effect.

Hydrotherapy

When one is under stress, it is very relaxing to slide into a warm or hot bathtub. The muscles quickly start to relax, deep regular breathing begins, and the cares that have been causing tension seem to float away with the steam. For centuries people have found this simple, accessible therapy extremely helpful as well as enjoyable.

Aromatherapy

Adding aromatic oils to the bathtub gives an even more beneficial effect. Try ylang-ylang, geranium, rose, neroli, melissa, lavender, sandalwood, or patchouli.

Herbal therapy

- Cardamom, peppermint, and fennel aid digestion and clear gas and bloating.
- Chamomile, rosemary, and lemon balm will help to soothe away the tension that can causes stomach upsets.
- Ginger will help to relieve acid reflux and heartburn.
- Meadowsweet and marshmallow are effective for an inflamed stomach lining with stomachache.
- Peppermint aids digestion and settles the stomach.
- Slippery elm soothes the stomach lining and eases acid indigestion.

Stress management

Stressful situations have a direct effect on the stomach lining, producing inflammation and resultant symptoms. So it is very important to look at lifestyle issues, such as interpersonal relationships and work situations, where a high proportion of stress occurs. Often changes made in these areas ease tensions in the body and troublesome symptoms diminish.

Massage

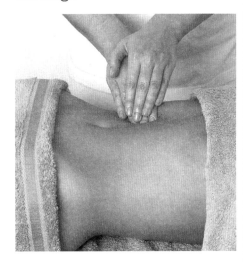

Place the fingertips of one hand on top of those of your other hand. Follow the direction of the large intestine with careful petrissage strokes.

Meditation

With indigestion, it is important to be able to achieve a state of calmness. This can best be accomplished by finding the method most suitable for you for gaining access to the refreshing stillness that exists at the center of each of us. It is useful to develop this ability when feeling well, so that you can carry it out at times of stress and illness.

Geranium essential oil is one of many that can be added to a bath to help release tension.

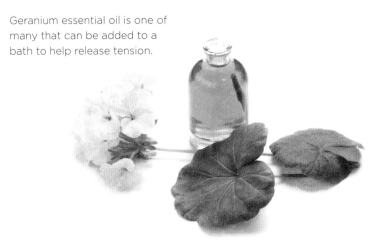

SEE ALSO

Symptoms

- Chest pain page 56
- Abdominal pain page 78
- Anxiety and panic page 130
- Depression page 134
- Eating disorders page 142
- Symptoms relating to immune function page 166

Therapies

- Reflexology page 195
- Therapeutic touch page 212
- Imagery page 218
- Homeopathy page 244
- Combating environmental pollution page 248

JAUNDICE

Jaundice is a yellowish diffuse discoloration of the skin and the whites of the eyes. It indicates the failure of the liver and biliary tract to excrete bile adequately into the intestinal tract, thence to be eliminated from the body. In its more advanced form, it may be associated with a pungent odor to the breath, itching of the skin, a brownish color of the urine, and light-colored stools.

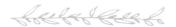

Conventional Therapies

- Bed rest, fluids, and simple foods
- Palliative treatment, such as removal of fluid from the abdomen
- Surgery

The causes of jaundice may be inside or outside the liver. In the liver the situation may be acute, as in hepatitis, or chronic, as in cirrhosis or scarring of the liver substance. Outside the liver the cause is usually obstructive, as in a tumor pressing against the biliary tract or a gallstone lodged in the bile duct.

COMPLEMENTARY THERAPIES
Diet and nutrition
Optimal nutrition is essential to the healing of any disturbance of the liver. This often creates a dilemma, because loss of appetite is common in liver inflammation.

- A strong program of vitamin–mineral supplementation is essential with liver conditions, because appetite and food intake are reduced.

- Extremely high levels of vitamins and minerals in liver and kidney disease may cause a buildup of nutrients in the body due to impaired excretion. A good rule of thumb might be to use only half the amounts usually considered optimal until the crisis is past and the liver shows clear signs of having resumed functioning.

Exercise
It is a good general rule with any liver condition to restrict physical activity to a minimum. However, with the passage of time, a dilemma arises because with prolonged physical inactivity come a number of negative effects—muscle deconditioning and wasting, weakness, further loss of appetite, etc. In this situation, it is a good idea to flex the arms and legs at regular intervals to help preserve joint mobility and stimulate circulation.

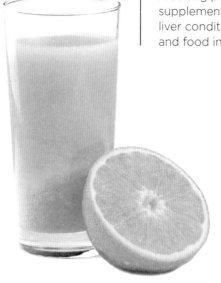

Fresh fruit and plenty of fluids are recommended in jaundice and may tempt a flagging appetite.

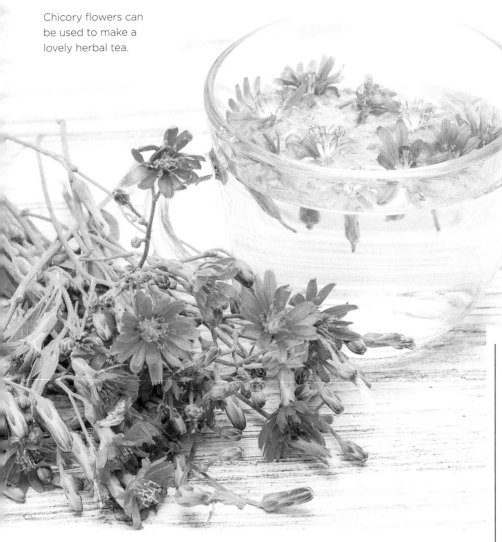

Chicory flowers can be used to make a lovely herbal tea.

SEE ALSO

Symptoms

- Infections page 50

- Fatigue page 52

- Abdominal pain page 78

- Addictions page 138

Therapies

- Reflexology page 195

- Acupressure page 200

- Imagery page 218

- Group therapy page 223

- Homeopathy page 244

Herbal therapy

- Alder buckthorn bark (1 part), restharrow root (5 parts), yellow gentian root (5 parts), and peppermint leaves (10 parts)—steep 1 teaspoon in 1/2 cup boiling water. Take 1–1 1/2 cups a day, in mouthful doses.

- Alder buckthorn bark (1 part), woodruff (2 parts), rosemary flowers (3 parts), and celadine (6 parts)—steep 2 teaspoons in 1/2 cup boiling water. Take 1/2 cup before breakfast and 1/2 cup at bedtime, in mouthful doses on each occasion.

- Chicory flowers (1 part), woodruff (1 part), dandelion root (2 parts), and speedwell (2 parts)—steep 1 teaspoon in 1/2 cup boiling water. Take 1 cup a day in mouthful doses, unsweetened.

DIABETIC SYMPTOMS

Questions sometimes arise concerning hidden cases of diabetes. A person may not be quite up to par and there may be a family history of diabetes, all of which can cause worry and concern.

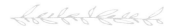

Conventional Therapies

- Diet, with calorie restriction and reduction of fats and starches
- Oral drugs
- Injection of insulin to control blood sugar

The truth of the matter is that at the earliest definable stage there may be no symptoms pointing to diabetes. It is not uncommon for the condition to be exposed by a coincidental infection, leading to symptoms such as excessive appetite and thirst and urination, in the presence of general weakness and even weight loss. If these symptoms occur, you should seek medical help, since there are one or two other possibilities that need to be ruled out. Action can be taken at home when blood sugar tests are in the borderline range between normal and abnormal. This is the ideal time to try to reset the trend back toward normal and keep it there.

In the largest category of patients—those who do not require insulin—the tendency to diabetes can be held at bay indefinitely with the proper attention. When diabetes has been present for a number of years, the situation may be entirely different and the well-known complications may have begun to appear. These include visual problems, various problems with blood circulation, neuritis, and kidney failure. People with a tendency to diabetes have a great incentive to avoid these by taking good care of themselves.

COMPLEMENTARY THERAPIES
Diet and nutrition

The optimal nutrition program discussed in the Therapies section is a blueprint for avoiding diabetes, in terms of the quality of its content. Part of the profile of the potential diabetic is a tendency to be overweight. So it is very important to build weight control into the overall program, starting with a dietary approach for maximum benefit.

- Using tobacco products correlates with the development of diabetes. You may not think of smoking as part of nutrition, but it is part of the chemical–metabolic equation.
- Low levels of magnesium are found in the tissues of diabetics, so the intake of adequate amounts is important.

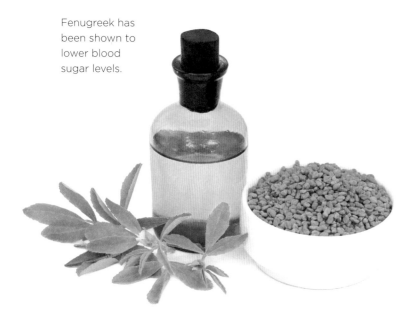

Fenugreek has been shown to lower blood sugar levels.

"When insulin is required to maintain blood sugar levels, even very young diabetics can learn how to administer injections to themselves."

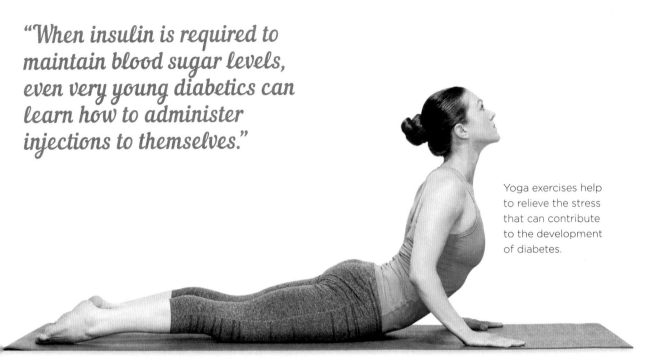

Yoga exercises help to relieve the stress that can contribute to the development of diabetes.

- Nicotinamide (niacin) may be useful in pre-diabetics, as it has been shown to preserve the integrity of the cells in the pancreas whose deterioration is responsible for diabetes.
- Vitamin E, evening primrose oil, and fish oil preparations are all beneficial in controlling blood sugar levels.
- Some studies suggest that vegetarian diets lower the risk of diabetes.
- In susceptible infants, cow's milk is 50 percent more likely than breast milk to lead to diabetes.

Exercise

A number of studies show strong evidence that exercise is an important factor in the avoidance of diabetes, both the insulin-dependent and the noninsulin-dependent types. If you are at risk (or even if you are not), choose the kind and amount of exercise that is most suitable for you and practice it on a regular basis.

Yoga

Certain yoga exercises, such as the Cobra shown above, are ideal ways of improving energy levels, which can often fall below normal in diabetics.

Herbal therapy

- Aloe is effective in lowering blood sugar.
- Fenugreek has been shown to lower blood sugar and urine sugar excretion.

Stress management

Stress has been shown to be a significant factor in the development of diabetes. It is a good idea to look into interpersonal relationships, both at home and at work, since this is where so many stress elements reside, and see how these situations might be improved.

SEE ALSO

Symptoms

- Dizziness page 36
- Infections page 50
- Fatigue page 52
- Loss of consciousness page 122
- Weight disorders page 146
- Intestinal symptoms page 160

Therapies

- Meditation page 215
- Homeopathy page 244

INTESTINAL SYMPTOMS

The intestinal part of the gastrointestinal tract is physiologically more important than the stomach. We can live without a stomach, but cannot live without an intestine. Most of the digestion, or breaking down, of food and most of the absorption of nutrients take place in the small intestine.

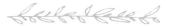

Conventional Therapies

- High-fiber diet
- Antispasmodic and pain-relieving drugs
- Anti-gas medications
- Anti-inflammatory drugs
- Laxatives and stool softeners
- Surgery

Briefly, digestion works like this. We chew our food and at the same time enzymes in the saliva act on it. Then it is swallowed into the stomach, where powerful acids and other enzymes break it down. The resulting acid emulsion (chyme) moves into the upper small intestine (the duodenum) to mix with the alkaline secretions of the liver, pancreas, and intestinal glands. These secretions contain powerful enzymes that split protein, carbohydrate, and fat fragments into smaller and smaller pieces, until they are tiny enough to pass through the wall of the intestine into the bloodstream, to be delivered to the body cells. Water moves freely back and forth between the intestine and the bloodstream to maintain the proper acidity and consistency of the intestinal contents.

The action of normal intestinal bacteria on the contents is another important part of the digestive process. When the contents move into the colon, enough water is removed to allow the formation of a solid mass, which is expelled from the body.

Many symptoms are caused by variations in the operation of this system, among which are the following.

Pain: This is largely due to spasm of the muscles of the intestine wall. This is experienced in acute inflammation, such as in viral gastroenteritis, ileitis, or colitis, and also irritable bowel syndrome, in which the normal rhythmic action of the intestinal muscles is disturbed by toxins, allergic reaction to foods, emotional influences, and so on.

Gas and bloating: These are generally due to faulty or incomplete digestion, with excessive gas production. A certain amount of intestinal gas is normal and increases a little with age, but when gas production is excessive, especially in the presence of intestinal spasm, cramping and bloating can occur. Deficiencies in the digestive process are often traceable to inadequate secretion of digestive enzymes, especially from the pancreas.

Constipation: This is a complex problem and can be due to one or more factors. Sluggish peristalsis (i.e. the contraction of the colon, which moves its contents) is one of the major causes. It is seen in poor general health, inactive elderly people, and in some low metabolic states, such as hypothyroidism and

"An allergic reaction to substances in cow's milk can be a cause of constipation in infants."

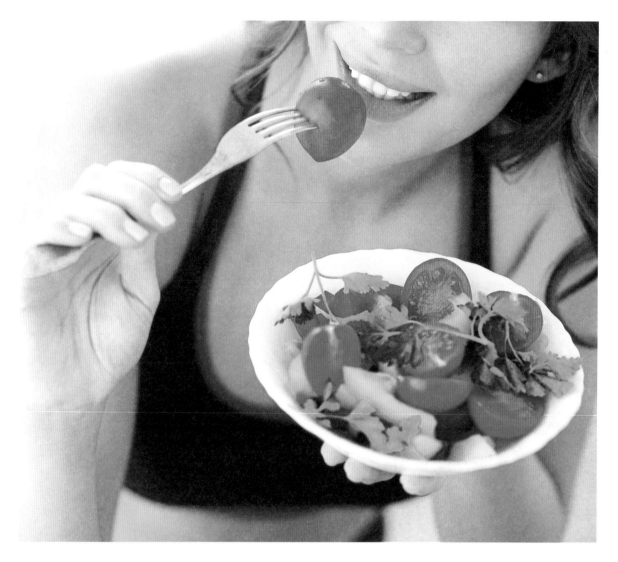

depression. The inability to relax the anal sphincter muscles is another. This is seen in states of anxiety and tension and often stems from childhood or adolescence, frequently lasting for years. Hard stools are also a common cause. They are the result of a combination of dietary factors (e.g. a high-meat, high-fat diet) and retention of feces in the colon for too long, resulting in the withdrawal of too much water from the fecal material.

Diarrhea: This common symptom of intestinal overactivity is the result of one or more of a number of factors. Infection, which can be generalized, as in the "flu" syndrome, or localized to the bowel, as in amebic dysentery, may be the cause. Food poisoning, the result of toxins liberated by the action of bacteria on spoiled food, is also a likely candidate. Metabolic conditions, including diabetes and hyperthyroidism, can produce serious prolonged diarrhea.

There are also two well-known syndromes that feature diarrhea as a symptom. Irritable bowel syndrome, a chronic low-level disturbance that can manifest all of the symptoms we are describing in this section, is believed to be due to a combination of

Fiber, vitamins, and minerals from fresh fruit and vegetables are the keys to intestinal health.

inappropriate food, psychological influences, food intolerance, antibiotic use, and previous infections. Inflammatory bowel disease is probably related to the auto-immune mechanisms, including regional enteritis, Crohn's disease, and ulcerative colitis. These conditions are potentially serious, capable of causing disability and death.

Flatulence: The passage of gas via the rectum is a normal phenomenon. Flatulence is a self-defined condition— "gas" becomes "flatulence" when it becomes malodorous and/or socially embarrassing. By and large, when the state of nutrition is good and the rectum is empty, intestinal gas will be produced virtually without odor.

COMPLEMENTARY THERAPIES
Diet and nutrition

In no area is it more important to adopt an optimal nutrition program than in intestinal problems. We have known for many years that diets low in fiber produce small, hard stools, but beyond curing that, an optimal diet supplies much of what the body needs to be in balance, and most of the factors that produce bowel trouble are reduced in influence. Here are a few specifics.

- Psyllium husks are well-known for their ability to help the bowel toward normal function.
- Constipation and diarrhea are correlated with food sensitivities in a number of studies. It is necessary to engage in a food elimination program to pinpoint the offenders.
- Constipation in infants has been shown to be related to cow's milk allergy.
- Vitamin A has been used successfully to treat diarrhea in children.

Acupressure

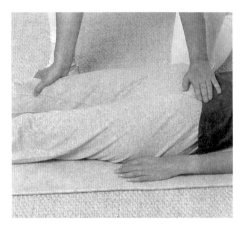

To treat diarrhea, place one comforting hand just below the navel and use the other to press the inside of each leg, about three fingers below the knee crease, in the groove behind the shin bone.

Reflexology

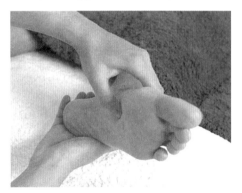

To relieve constipation, clear and balance the stomach and pancreas area by thumb-walking in three horizontal rows below the diaphragm (or protruding chest) reflex. Also work the intestines (see page 79). Combine with relaxing, nurturing movements to release locked emotion.

Imagery

Hypnotherapy has achieved excellent results in irritable bowel syndrome. Once this has proved effective, imagery and self-hypnosis can be practiced at home on a continuing basis to maintain the good effects of the hypnotherapy.

Biofeedback

Biofeedback training has been used with excellent results in chronic constipation, fecal incontinence, and irritable bowel syndrome, either alone or in combination with progressive relaxation and coping training.

Homeopathy

The following remedies have been of benefit in diarrhea: arsenicum album, chamomilla, mercurius vivua, podophyllum, and sulfur.

Herbal therapy

- Bayberry, agrimony, and comfrey root are good for diarrhea in adults.
- Chamomile and lemon balm will ease diarrhea.
- Licorice, ginger, dandelion root, yellow dock root, and burdock are effective for constipation.
- Meadowsweet is useful for upset stomach accompanied by diarrhea.
- Peppermint will help to control muscle contractions and discomfort.

Meditation

It is very helpful to incorporate meditative techniques into any program for the relief of intestinal symptoms. Find the method that suits you best and practice it daily when you are feeling well. The technique will then be available when you are experiencing symptoms.

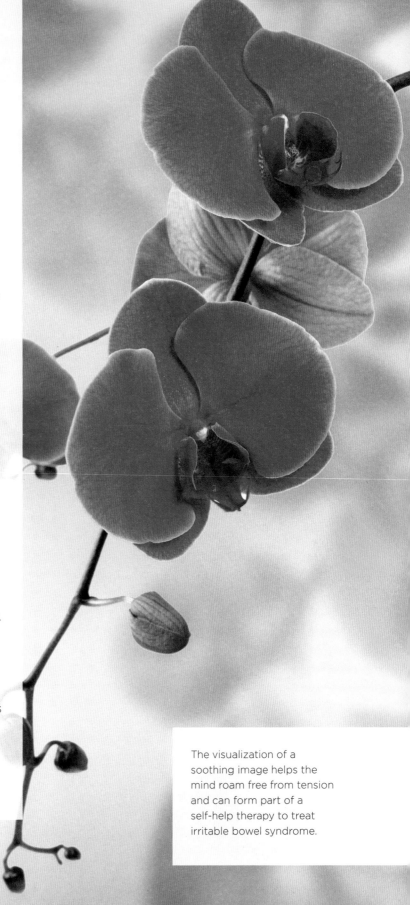

The visualization of a soothing image helps the mind roam free from tension and can form part of a self-help therapy to treat irritable bowel syndrome.

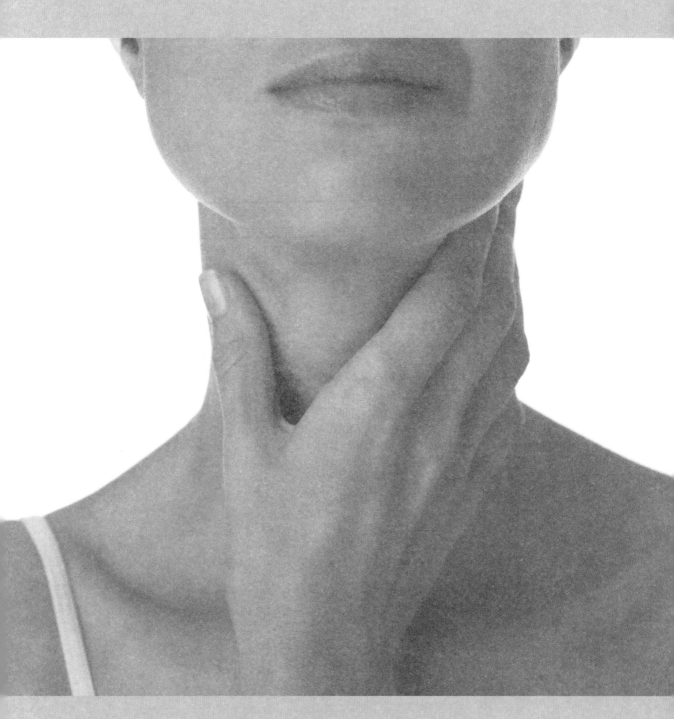

IMMUNE SYSTEM

SYMPTOMS RELATING TO IMMUNE FUNCTION

The immune system is one of the body's defense mechanisms. Its functions are to detect threats and to mobilize the body's defenses against them.

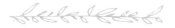

Conventional Therapies

■ Immunization

■ Suppression of activity of the immune system in a variety of diseases and in organ transplantation

The immune system has been under intense scrutiny over the past few decades because of its relevance both to certain immune disorders such as AIDS and to the field of organ transplantation. Many other areas are being explored, including hypersensitivity to many substances. This has led to a new field of exploration, called clinical ecology or environmental medicine.

The cells of the immune system include certain white blood cells and some related tissue cells. Most of these cells are produced in the bone marrow, liver, and spleen. Certain cells, identified as "helpers" and "suppressors" of immune responses, have the ability to attach themselves to other cells selectively, as a key fits a lock, thereby transferring certain active substances that can travel to various parts of the body at surprising speed.

As with all biological systems, a balance is required before the immune system can function optimally. In some people and situations the system is lazy or sluggish, not doing its job of repelling "invaders," while in others it is overly aggressive, producing needless inflammation, and even serious illness, in its own body. This has given rise to the designation autoimmune diseases.

The following are among the many symptoms relating to the immune system.

Allergic rhinitis: The recurrent stuffy nose is an indicator of many things, in the inhaled air, in food, and even in the emotional system.

Anaphylactic shock: This is the marked systemic reaction, fortunately uncommon, seen when the immune system goes into high gear in response to an external stimulus. It produces a total body response manifested by a drop in blood pressure, soft tissue swellings, difficulty in breathing, and alteration in consciousness, which can result in coma and death. The classic emergency treatment is adrenalin by injection, which works to neutralize the body's overreaction.

Asthma: This well-known condition is characterized by inadequate, wheezing respirations.

Autoimmune reaction: This happens when the body attacks itself with chemicals that can damage or destroy body tissues. Examples

"Rewarding physical exercise, at your own pace, helps the balanced working of the immune system."

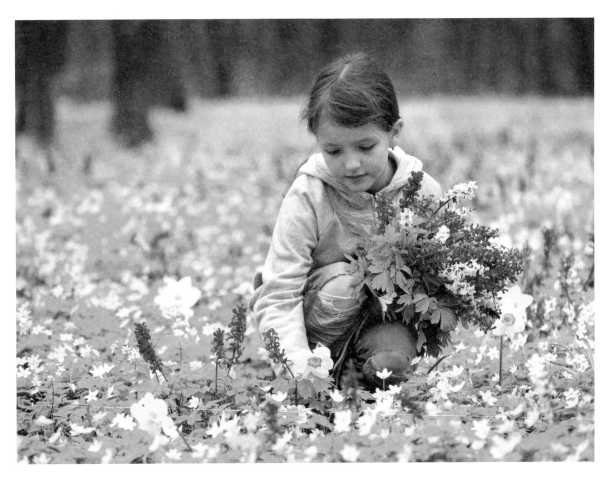

include severe rheumatoid arthritis, lupus, and spondylitis.

Food sensitivities: Only a few years ago, allergists denied that foods could produce allergies, largely because their testing methods were not broad enough. It is mainly clinical ecologists who have made these connections. Among the conditions found to be related to food sensitivity are atopic dermatitis, asthma, attention deficit disorder, hyperactivity in children, rheumatoid arthritis, fatigue, constipation, cardiac arrhythmia, bedwetting, hearing loss, migraine, multiple sclerosis, otitis media, and peptic ulcer.

Hay fever: This is one of the many airborne respiratory allergies that cause much distress and some serious illness.

Hives: Also called urticaria, this is a skin manifestation of a general systemic allergic reaction. It is important as a possible harbinger of a more serious subsequent reaction to the same stimulus.

HIV/AIDS: This condition, in which the immune system itself is attacked, spawns myriad symptoms, which are becoming better known to the public all the time. The subject of AIDS is already too vast to be covered here, but many of the complementary approaches outlined below are applicable.

Insect bites and stings: Some bites and stings are capable of leading to anaphylactic reactions and death.

Hay fever happens when antibodies in the nasal lining react to pollen.

COMPLEMENTARY THERAPIES
Herbal therapy

Astragalus, echinacea, eupatorium, licorice, chamomile, arnica, sylimarin, and Viscum album have been found effective in immune disorders.

Diet and nutrition

A host of studies in the past decade or so have measured the effects of substances on immune system functioning, giving rise to the following observations.

- Daily micronutrient intakes of the average older person are too low to support optimal immunity.
- Large doses of B vitamins diminish the adverse stress on the immune system.
- Lower fat intake has been demonstrated to improve immune function.
- Vitamin A increases immunity and decreases mortality in measles. In one study, 200,000 units daily for two days was shown to reduce the risk of death and major complications by 49 percent.
- Iron is involved in immunity; either overload or deficiency will compromise immune function.
- Selenium supplementation increases the activity of immune cells without changing selenium blood levels.

- Multivitamin supplementation in one large study correlated with a 50 percent reduction in days lost from work due to illness.
- Vitamins B, C, E, A, and beta-carotene, selenium, and zinc were found to enhance immune function.
- Melatonin (a naturally occurring substance) affects the immune system by modulating natural steroid release and zinc turnover to affect the immune cells. Melatonin and zinc taken together can restore full activity of thymic hormone production, strengthening the immune system.
- AIDS patients are deficient in folic acid in all stages of the illness.
- Routine vitamin/mineral supplementation in AIDS is cheaper than repeated testing for specific deficiencies.
- Calcium and zinc reduce nasal swelling in allergic rhinitis.
- Magnesium taken intravenously is very helpful in anaphylactic shock and severe asthma.
- Low intake of magnesium in a study of 2,400 people was shown to correlate with an increased risk of wheezing.
- Food sensitivity was found to be implicated in 25 percent of atopic dermatitis.
- Attention deficit disorder is correlated with the use of artificial flavors and colors, chocolate, caffeine, white sugar, and monosodium glutamate.
- Hyperactivity is similarly related. Steps in management include food recording, elimination of suspected foods, and then re-exposure to them.
- Rheumatoid arthritis correlates with food sensitivity in many studies.

Imagery

Allergies such as asthma have been helped by imagery techniques, which help to achieve desensitization and the reduction of stress.

The controlled use of bee stings has proved effective in treating some immune disorders.

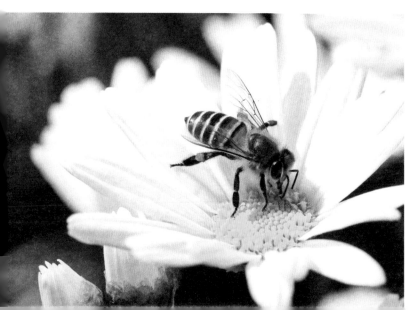

Bee venom therapy

This therapy has been used with success in many immune disorders, including autoimmune diseases. In this therapy, which has a long history of documented success, the use of bee stings under controlled conditions has been shown to modify the immune system response in autoimmune diseases, causing improvement in the symptoms of conditions that include lupus and rheumatoid arthritis.

The controlled use of bee stings has proved effective in treating some immune disorders.

Exercise

Aerobic exercise has been shown to increase specific immune cells. Daily exercise within your capabilities is important for the maintenance of immune function. Running and swimming, practiced with the correct breathing, can help respiratory allergies.

Breathing therapy

Practicing a breathing and relaxation program suitable for you can help to boost the immune system and is usefully supplemented by massage and therapeutic touch, especially in the case of AIDS.

Stress management

Stress has been shown to compromise the immune system, among many other functions of the body. Examine carefully those things that you know or suspect produce stress in your life, especially your relationships at home and at work, which are always such prominent stress-generators.

Bach flower remedies

- Beech (food intolerance)
- Clematis (oversensitivity)
- Impatiens (skin irritation and hay fever)
- Mimulus (fear of oncoming illness in HIV/AIDS)

Acupressure

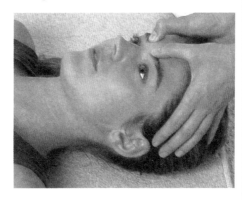

For hay fever relief, press bladder point 2, located on the inside edges of the eyebrows where the hair is thickest.

Massage

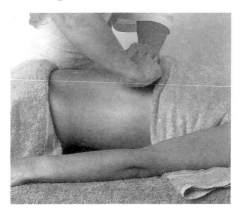

Combat breathing difficulties by tracing horizontally across the ribs under the breast with a loose fist, using the back of the knuckles. This helps to free the intercostal muscles between the ribs, so that the rib cage can swing easily up and out for unrestricted breathing.

Meditation

The ability to make regular connection with the calm center of one's being has a direct bearing on the balances of the body. The equilibrium of the immune system is one of the most important.

SEE ALSO

Symptoms

- Swollen glands page 42
- Infections page 50
- Joint pain page 94
- Skin symptoms page 104

Therapies

- Hydrotherapy page 231
- Homeopathy page 244

AGING

The story of the complex process of aging is constantly being rewritten. The life-expectancy tables of just a generation ago have been completely revised and the trend to longer life shows no sign of diminishing.

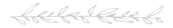

SEE ALSO

■ All the symptoms and therapies discussed in this book have some bearing on the various processes and concepts of aging.

However, a long life brings a number of potential problems: longer-lasting financial pressures; insufficient rewarding activity and long hours to fill; the specter of degenerative diseases; and possible prolonged dependency on others. This litany of disaster would be quite depressing if it were not for the fact that a strategy exists to lessen the impact of each of these undeniable problem areas.

Aging of the body tissues occurs when the normal process of replacing a worn-out cell with a fresh one is not carried out properly. This faulty copying process is caused in large part by a process called oxidation, which is due to a combination of factors, as follows:

■ Environmental influences play a major role, including contaminants in our food, in the air we breathe, in radiation and ultraviolet rays, and probably emotional stress.

■ Disease processes, such as fatty degeneration of tissues and autoimmune diseases, many of which are traceable to the environmental factors above, are another issue.

■ There are also intrinsic body reactions in the eventual winding down of body processes.

Many of the substances that combat oxidation occur naturally in the body, but they are often insufficient at times of metabolic stress. Others come from sources, including vitamins C and E, that are discussed elsewhere in this book, especially under Diet and Nutrition in the Therapies section.

An optimal nutrition program, combined with daily exercise and a positive state of mind, is the best way to retard the aging process. Relaxation therapies, such as meditation, imagery, yoga, and tai chi, are found especially beneficial in promoting this sense of harmony and "wellness."

Attitude and Planning

Our thinking about aging should be positive, based on the "can do" attitude adopted during our primary career.

■ Try to develop stimulating, sustainable activities during the career years. Have a list of "things I have always wanted to do"—and do them!

■ Put thought and effort into making as much financial provision as possible.

■ Maintain health and well-being—a lifelong pursuit to be continued with equal vigor in the later years.

"*Planning and a positive attitude can make the later years a time of rewarding activity.*"

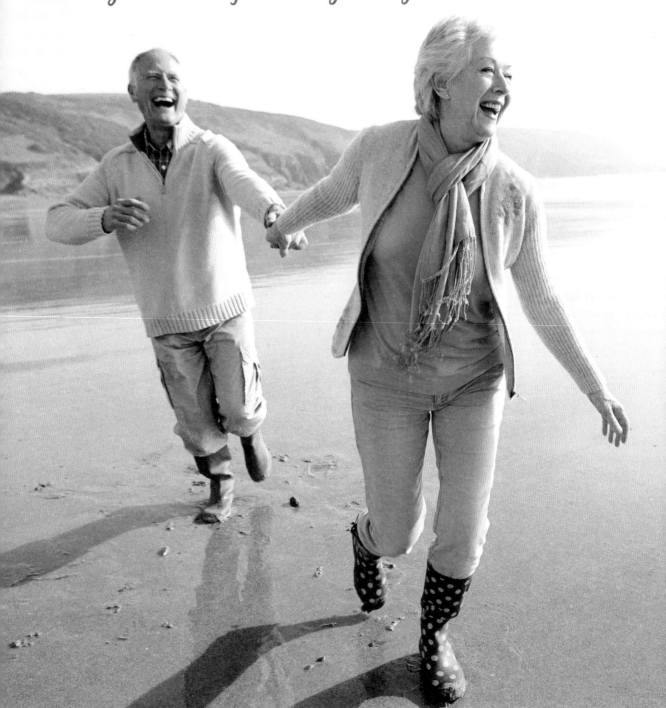

THERAPIES

This section gives you more detailed information about complementary and alternative therapies, and how they can help you to treat specific symptoms in the way that works best for you. It also offers you a means to counter future illness and to achieve positive, lasting gains in the quality of your health and well-being.

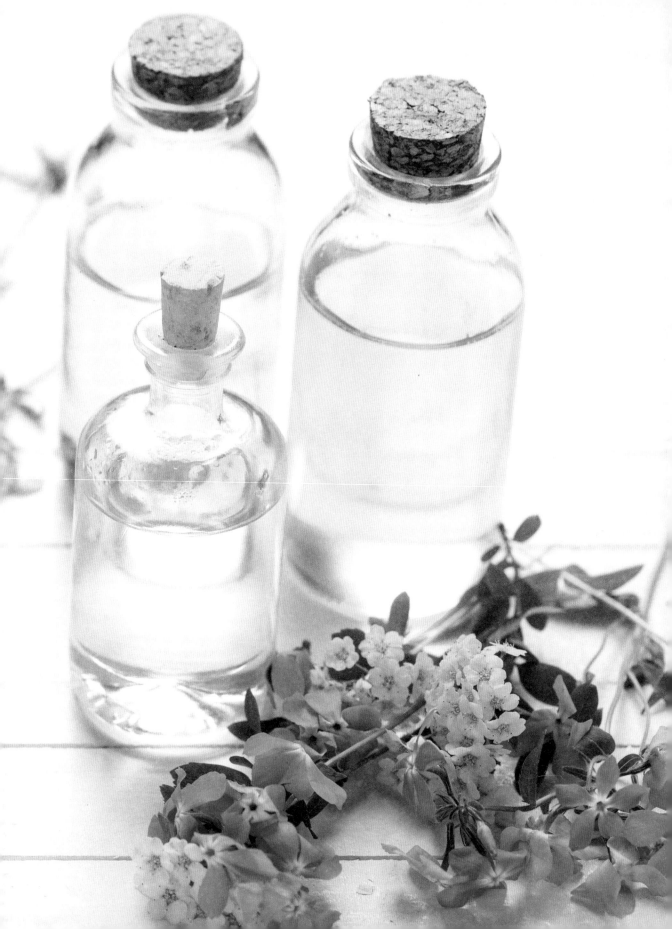

THERAPIES RELATING TO THE BODY AND ITS FUNCTIONS

These therapies approach our being by direct application to the physical structure of the body and the physiological processes taking place there. They have to do with the processes of digestion, respiration, and muscle action.

DIET AND NUTRITION

The food we eat is a cornerstone of good health, which is why so many of the symptoms refer to this section. An enormous amount has been written on the subject and many statements are controversial and/or contradictory. This book intends to be as clear and concise as possible, and to give the most useful information.

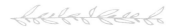

A healthy diet is relatively low in animal fats and high in fiber. Red meat and preserved meats should be eaten sparingly. Eggs need not be severely limited, since they are a healthy food. Research tells us that margarine is not a healthy food—see Better Butter on page 176 for a healthy alternative. Cheese should not be eaten with reckless abandon, though it is all right in moderation. Adults do not need much milk, so a good practice is to buy low-fat milk for tea or coffee and for use in cooking, and drink it sparingly. Avoid fizzy drinks as they contain many artificial substances.

Whole grains are valuable in the diet both for their fiber content and the many nutrients they contain. Good sources are cereals (with a minimum of additives and sweeteners) and baked goods. There are many bakeries now that bake single and multigrain breads; those who are allergic to wheat can usually find good alternatives there, such as rice, oat, and rye breads. Even the old art of home baking is making a comeback!

To sweeten food, where necessary, use honey, natural syrups (e.g. maple), and less refined, unbleached sugars (e.g. demerara) instead of refined sugar and artificial sweeteners. It is important that your food be fresh, so shop often and discard food before it spoils. It is especially important to avoid rancid fats and oils. Eat lots of fresh fruits, salads, and vegetables of all kinds, cooking the latter lightly. Healthy salad oils, such as canola and safflower, should not be used in stir-frying, because they are altered by the extreme heat. Instead, use a stable oil like olive oil, with perhaps just a touch of butter for its flavor.

Adding herbs to food is a very healthy practice, and enhances and varies the flavor of food enormously. The day of dull cooked vegetables is definitely over, once you learn to cook your vegetables lightly and add these delicious seasonings.

These foods not only look delicious but also have the nutrients to do you good.

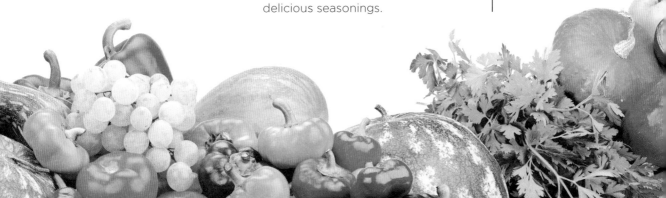

Have a Heart-healthy Day!

Breakfast

- ½ grapefruit or 1 fresh orange (fresh fruit with pulp is better for you than juice alone)—fresh berries in summer are an excellent alternative!

- Two slices of oatmeal or other whole-grain toast, spread lightly with Better Butter

- A modest bowl of granola muesli can substitute for toast. Avoid the sweetened, processed varieties, and add 2% milk if desired

- 1 cup of fresh ground, filtered coffee or 1 cup of tea, regular or herbal. Sweeten with a scant teaspoonful of honey and add 2% or skim milk if desired

Lunch in winter

- A bowl of hearty homemade soup, such as vegetable, leek and potato, or mushroom, or a corn or fish chowder

- A small tuna and celery salad with a few slices of almond and low-fat mayonnaise. Season with herbs (e.g. dill, parsley, cilantro)

- An occasional alternative: an egg salad with herbs and watercress

- A slice of whole-grain bread, or a muffin or roll, spread with almond butter if desired

- A piece of fresh fruit for dessert if desired

Lunch in summer

- Fresh garden salad or fruit salad—if you like cold soups, the following can be tasty and nourishing:
Chilled gazpacho
Tomato seasoned with herbs and a dash of orange juice
Cold leek and potato
Chilled consommé

- A slice of good bread or a salad sandwich if you are not worried about overdoing the bread!

- Plain natural yogurt over fresh fruit is a summer lunch treat

Dinner

- Zucchini quiche (no crust) or vegetable lasagna or baked or broiled fish with herbs

- Fresh broccoli with lemon

- Herbed rice or parsleyed boiled potatoes

- Tomato halves baked with crumbs, parsley, and garlic and drizzled with olive oil (these go well with the fish or the zucchini quiche)

- Dessert, if desired:
Individual baked custards
Stewed fruit with yogurt

Better butter

Leave 1lb (450g) of butter at room temperature until it becomes softened (not to the point of melting). Use lightly salted, unsalted, or a combination of the two. Cut the butter into chunks and place in a food processor. Beat in a scant cup (250ml) of canola oil (or safflower or sunflower if you prefer). When the oil and butter are well mixed and smooth, put into small crocks, cover, and either freeze or put in the refrigerator. Better Butter keeps well. Whenever it becomes too soft at room temperature, just firm it up in the refrigerator. It has half the animal fat of butter and is tasty, spreadable, and unadulterated by the addition of substances the body does not recognize as food.

Use the Better Butter recipe above to make a mixture with good taste and spreadability, but with half the animal fat of butter.

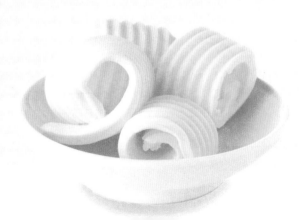

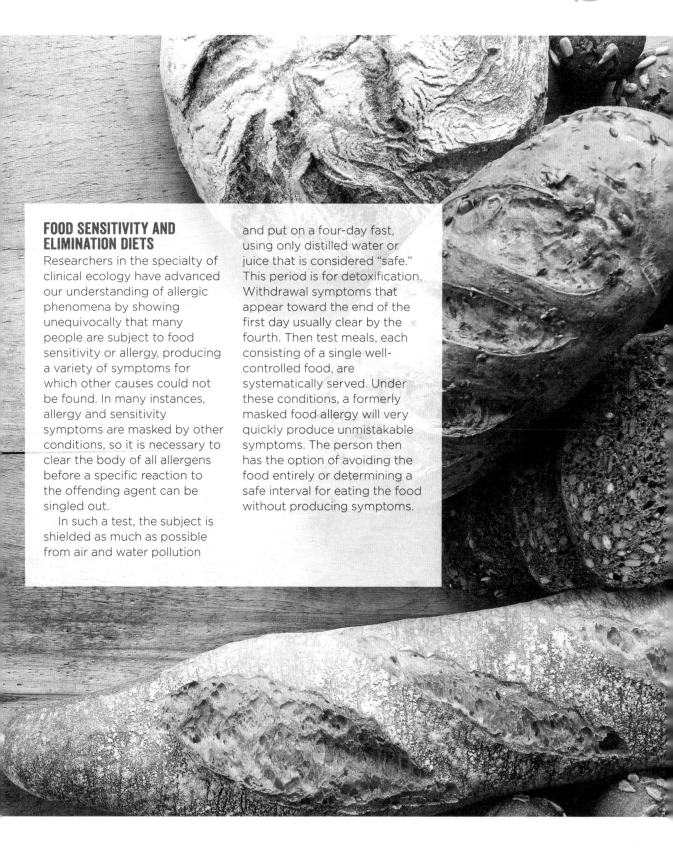

FOOD SENSITIVITY AND ELIMINATION DIETS

Researchers in the specialty of clinical ecology have advanced our understanding of allergic phenomena by showing unequivocally that many people are subject to food sensitivity or allergy, producing a variety of symptoms for which other causes could not be found. In many instances, allergy and sensitivity symptoms are masked by other conditions, so it is necessary to clear the body of all allergens before a specific reaction to the offending agent can be singled out.

In such a test, the subject is shielded as much as possible from air and water pollution and put on a four-day fast, using only distilled water or juice that is considered "safe." This period is for detoxification. Withdrawal symptoms that appear toward the end of the first day usually clear by the fourth. Then test meals, each consisting of a single well-controlled food, are systematically served. Under these conditions, a formerly masked food allergy will very quickly produce unmistakable symptoms. The person then has the option of avoiding the food entirely or determining a safe interval for eating the food without producing symptoms.

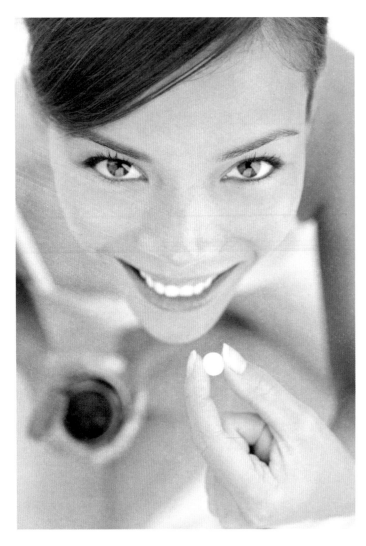

Regular intake of selected vitamins and minerals can help prevent illness and fight pain.

NUTRITIONAL SUPPLEMENTS

An older school of thought asserts that you can get all the nutrients you need from your food, but a wealth of research and experience now contradicts that point of view, on a number of grounds, including lack of information available to the consumer, unavailability of an ideal balance of foods at any given time, exhaustion of the soil by profit-driven, large-scale farming, and degradation of the food chain with toxic products. From this knowledge, plus the realization that there are many more nutritional deficiencies than were previously known, it is clear that adequate nutrition depends upon the addition of various supplements to our diet. The research in this area is extensive and the use of supplements has been shown to relieve, and even prevent, many symptoms of illness. These nutritional supplements include vitamins, minerals, and various other substances.

The word "vitamin" comes from "vital amine," meaning a nitrogen-containing substance that is essential to life. This is agreed upon by all, but what is not agreed is the amount of each vitamin necessary for sparkling good health. The Recommended Dietary Allowances (RDA) were put out in 1974 by the National Research Council (not to be confused with the USRDA used by the Food and Drug Administration for nutritional labeling) and some of the levels have occasionally been updated according to more recent information. The basis for using these levels is either by determining the level below which a specific deficiency disease will occur or, in the absence of that kind of information, by determining the average intake of a substance by an apparently healthy group of volunteers. In recent years the concept of optimal health has developed to denote vigorous, vibrant health at all levels of activity, as opposed to the antiquated concept of health as merely the absence of disease. In an effort to define the level of nutritional support that will enable optimal health functioning, a number of authors in the nutritional field have published data on their clinical experience, including the levels of dietary supplements they have found to be supportive of optimal health. The level of vitamins and other supplements shown here can be taken safely on a daily basis and will enhance your experience of life. It should be noted that the amounts recommended

Daily Supplements for Optimal Health

Vitamins	Optimal levels*	Units	US RDA
Beta-carotene	25,000	IU	6,000
Vitamin B1	100	mg	1.5
Vitamin B2	100	mg	1.7
Niacin	100	mg	1.0
Vitamin B6	50	mg	2.0
Vitamin B12	50	meg	2.0xq
Folic acid	400	meg	200
Vitamin C	2,000–6,000	mg	60
Vitamin D	400 or less	IU	200
Vitamin E	400–800	IU	200
Minerals			
Calcium	500–1,000	mg	800
Magnesium	250–500	mg	350
Selenium	200–400	mg	70
Zinc	15–30	mg	15
Other nutrients			
Coenzyme Q	60–100	mg	—
EPA (eicosapentaenoic acid)	180–270	mg	—
DHA (docosahexaenoic acid)	120–360	mg	—
Evening primrose oil	500	mg	—

* See page 256 for sources of author's recommendations.
IU = internal unit; mg = milligram; mcg = microgram

here are above USRDA levels, but they are well below levels that could be considered toxic or dangerous. These amounts can be varied by 10–15 percent without producing any significant difference to the body.

Most of the nutrients on the list have antioxidant properties—that is, they have the ability to oppose the body's natural tendency to oxidize chemical constituents in the body to produce toxic and other harmful substances. Nutritional biochemists assert that antioxidants work against the development of coronary artery disease, cancer, arthritis, and other diseases. This very important field is being studied intensively and new insights are continually emerging.

The topic of cholesterol continues to be in the news. As more people have become aware of the importance of separating HDL and LDL cholesterol, and of knowing what affects each, they have made progress in understanding cholesterol and its role in artery diseases.

The licensing of olestra, a fat substitute, by the FDA made headlines in the 1990s. This substance not only floats through the body unabsorbed, bringing unpleasant symptoms with it, but also absorbs the essential fat-soluble vitamins A, D, E, and K and carries them away as well.

For optimal results, it is a good idea to seek the advice of a nutritional therapist before selecting a course of supplements.

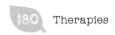

EXERCISE

Aerobic exercise is simply exercise that can be performed using energy created by the oxygen supply from the lungs, as in walking vigorously over a distance. When the oxygen supply of a muscle is exceeded, as in a short sprint, anaerobic metabolism comes into play, with energy produced by the conversion of glucose by glycolosis. The latter method of obtaining energy is only about 1/20th as efficient as aerobic energy production.

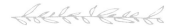

Jogging can be useful exercise, provided you do not overstress your joints or push yourself to the point of pain.

Exercise is very beneficial if done in the right way and for the right reasons. These are three good reasons for taking exercise.

- It conditions the muscles, including the heart muscle, with relatively short periods of intense effort. What the muscles need is an intense burst that really challenges the muscle cells to increase their output ability. This can be done with 10 minutes on a skiing or rowing machine every day or every other day. (An inexpensive rig will do the job.) The main caution is the effect on existing heart disease—consult your physician if in doubt. There is a lot of individual variation of opinion as to what quantity of exercise is beneficial.

- It controls the amount of fat the body carries around, and to some extent the composition of that fat. This can be most effectively pursued in conjunction with a healthy diet program. There is evidence to suggest that most forms of exercise stimulate the production of HDL cholesterol, aiding the health of the arteries.

- It helps you to achieve a sense of well-being. This can be done with a wide variety of exercise. Selection of the right type for this purpose is a matter of individual preference. While one person would like to perform light dance routines, another would prefer to take a brisk walk and another 20 minutes of wood chopping.

Eastern traditions, such as Ayurvedic medicine, place much emphasis on different body types and temperaments in the selection of exercise activities, though certain yoga practices, such as the Sun Salute, are suitable for everyone.

Jogging is a very popular practice in America, where many cities have jogging trails. While jogging doubtless gives satisfaction to those who perform it, there is some controversy as to how much it benefits health. Some argument centers around the effects of such long-sustained activity on the ligaments and joints, especially if done on hard surfaces. Always wear suitable shoes and socks, warm up first, and jog at a comfortable pace.

"Pace and grade your activities. Slow down or stop if you feel you are doing too much or going too fast."

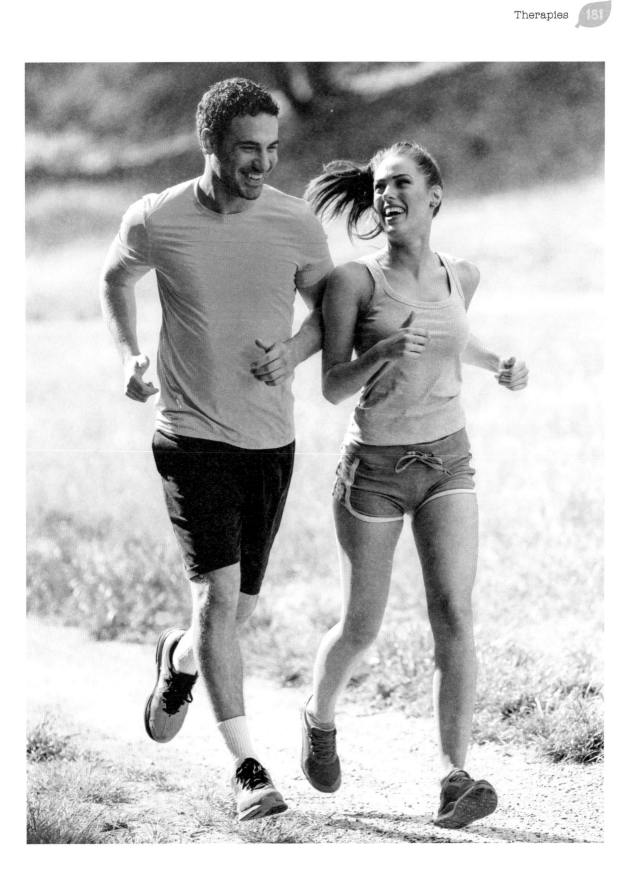

Being aware of your body and knowing when to stop exercising is just as important as knowing when to up the pace.

The best ways to assess the level of exercise that is right for you include the following.

- Listen to your body. Be aware of how your body is responding to the activity you have in mind. You are the only one who can detect the first signs of overuse. Watch for pain or aching in the chest or back, excessive breathlessness, dizziness, and weakness. Never ignore such warning signs.

- Pace and grade your activities. Slow down or stop if you feel you are doing too much or going too fast. Get the feel of doing just a little more in the next session of activity and keep going in this way until you reach whatever goal you have set for yourself.

- Have your body tested. If you have a serious doubt about whether your body is sound or should be pushed a little farther, do not hesitate to have yourself tested, either at a medical facility or a reliable fitness facility.

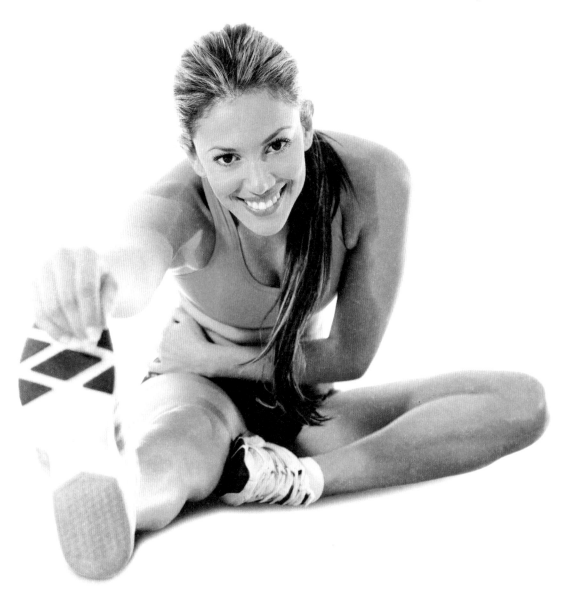

Basic Warm-up and Cool-down Routine

1 Raise the right shoulder while the left drops. Then raise the left and drop the right. Do this four times.

2 Drop your head toward your right shoulder, then toward your left. Repeat four times.

3 Swing your arms out as you jump and land with feet apart. Jump again, arms down and feet together.

4 Brings hands up in front of chest with arms rounded.

Press upper back away from hands for 10 seconds.

5 Clasp hands behind back with arms slightly bent. Squeeze shoulder blades tightly together for 10 seconds.

6 Straighten one leg, bend the other, and lean forward. Support weight on bent leg. Do 15 seconds with each leg.

7 Bend one leg and hold ankle. Keep knees level and push forward with hips. Do 15 seconds with each leg.

8 Put weight on front leg. Keep back toes pointing forward and heel on floor (A). Bring back leg forward and transfer weight to back leg (B). Hold both positions for 10 seconds with each leg.

9 Finish off with a full-body stretch.

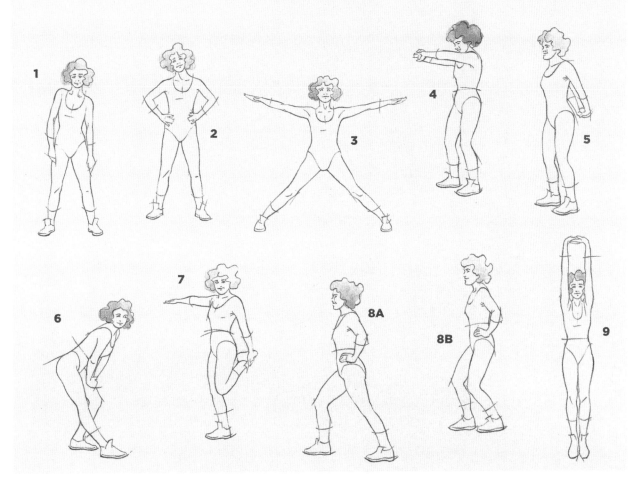

DANCE AND MOVEMENT

Dance and other activities involving body movement are often overlooked in the context of healing and wellness therapies, but they are powerful members of that group and have strong connections with body, mind, emotions, and spirit.

Dance of many different kinds is not only enjoyable exercise, but can also be valuable therapy in terms of bodily coordination, self-expression, and artistic pleasure.

Dance comes most naturally to those with a lean and strong body structure and a tendency to good coordination. As therapy, dance and movement are available and helpful to all. As the tactile and kinesthetic senses are involved, it is very useful for people whose movement and coordination are impaired as a result of damage to the nervous system.

Beyond this, dance and movement are helpful in the development of balance and coordination, self-confidence, and body awareness. When pursued to its ultimate heights, dance as an art form provides both the dancer and those who partake of his or her art with a sublime spiritual experience.

Increasingly, dance and movement are coming to be recognized as therapeutic on many levels of our being. Many more performances and workshops are becoming available, which demonstrates their value in terms of both art and therapy.

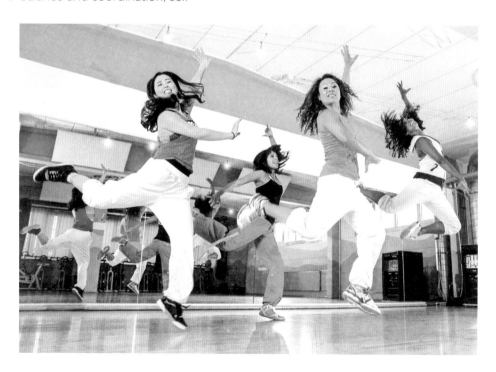

ALEXANDER TECHNIQUE

Named after F. Matthias Alexander, who developed it in the early 20th century, this is a practical technique based on body mechanics and balance. It is applied to the simple things we do every day, such as moving and breathing, eating and speaking, lifting and carrying, reading and writing.

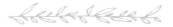

The technique must be learned from a qualified instructor and as many as 30 individual sessions may be required. By using hand contact, the teacher gives the student a new experience of coordination in carrying out everyday activities, showing the person that there are choices in how action is carried out. The teacher uses speech to connect "mental" choices to "physical" actions, demonstrating in practice that there is no separation between mind and body. Alexander said that "you translate everything, whether physical, mental, or spiritual, into muscular tension." The beneficial effects include improved breathing, reduced muscular pain and spasm, a protective effect on the internal organs, and an aura of self-confidence leading to physical and social grace. The technique makes possible levels of achievement and satisfaction that were formerly unattainable.

The Alexander technique can be reinforced at home by self-awareness and continued application until the newly acquired balances become automatic, bringing lifelong benefit. A series of sessions with a qualified instructor will gradually lead to a program of self-directed activities at home.

Alexander technique lessons are based around everyday activities and movements, such as sitting, standing, and walking, and basically help you to use your body without being so badly affected by the stresses and tension of living.

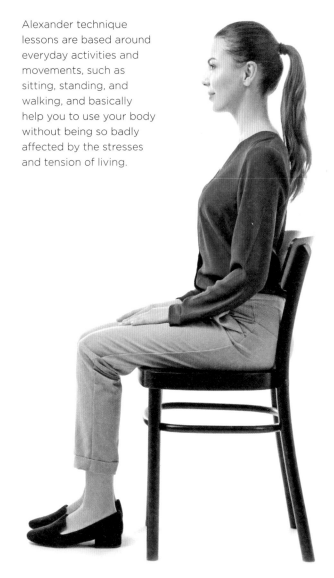

MASSAGE

Massage includes many different kinds and varieties of therapy. The word "massage" comes from the Greek word *massein*, meaning "to knead." There are references to the Chinese system of massage as early as 3000 B.C. Greek writing shows Hippocrates discussing the benefits of massage and this tradition was carried down the corridors of time, through Aesculapius, Celsus, the great Galen, and the Middle Ages in unbroken continuity to modern times.

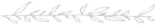

Most forms of massage techniques today work on certain soft tissues of the body, in particular the muscles, ligaments, and tendons. One of the purposes of massage is to induce relaxation, both in the structures being massaged and in the individual as a whole.

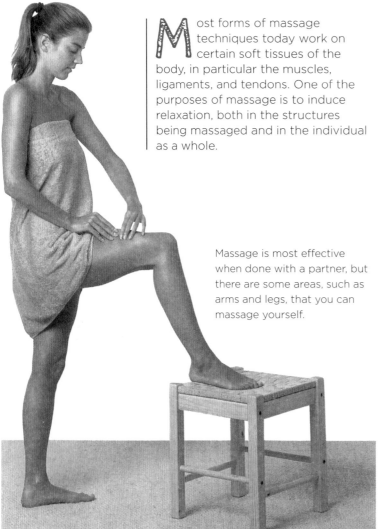

Massage is most effective when done with a partner, but there are some areas, such as arms and legs, that you can massage yourself.

Muscular relaxation is achieved by kneading the muscle tissue through the skin, especially in the regions of the neck, shoulders, and back. In these areas, underlying bony structures provide something against which to compress the muscle tissue. One learns how much pressure to exert to produce the desired effect. It takes only a little experience to begin to detect areas of tightness and spasm in a muscle. The massage serves to bring more blood into the area (and with it warmth), and in some instances one can feel the breaking up of small firm deposits, possibly the debris of metabolic processes within the muscle.

There are only certain areas of the body that one can massage for oneself—neck, shoulders, arms, legs, and feet—but even these are difficult, as muscles being massaged should be relaxed. Two people working together can reach areas that one person cannot, and the subject to be massaged can be positioned so that the muscles can relax fully.

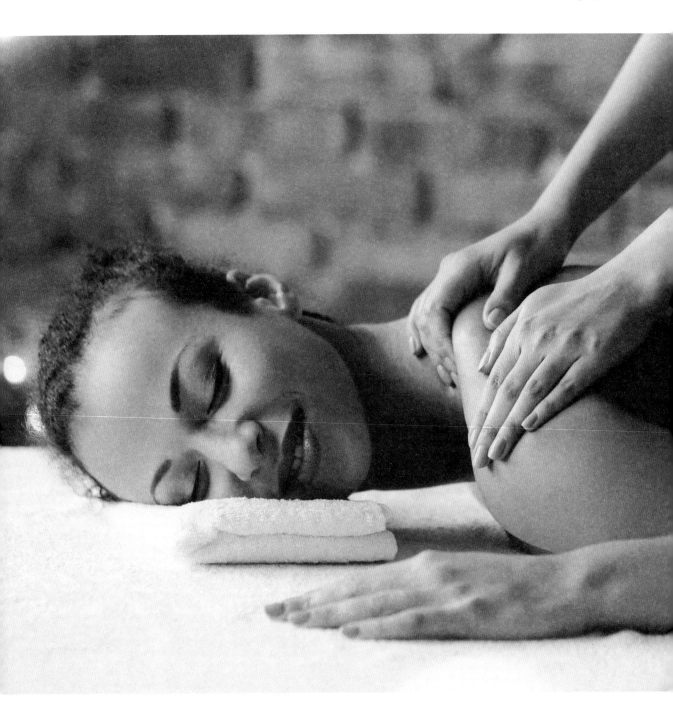

"Two people working together can reach areas that one person cannot, and the subject to be massaged can be positioned so that the muscles can relax fully."

In terms of the overall relaxation of the subject, it is clearly an advantage to work in pairs, so that the subject can be allowed to relax completely. The mechanisms of this relaxation involve a combination of physical, mental, emotional, and spiritual factors, which result from being in a warm space filled with soft, soothing music and a pleasant aroma, in which a friendly and sympathetic helper is present.

No verbal description of massage technique is as helpful as hands-on experience. This experience can be obtained in several ways.

- Learn from a friend who is already experienced.
- Find a massage therapist near you who is willing to spend some time to give you the necessary tips to use for your self-massage program.
- Attend a course to give you information and offer you hands-on experience.

"The effectiveness of massage lies in stimulating blood flow, relaxing nerves and muscles, and in the psychological benefits of feeling cared for."

Basic Massage Strokes

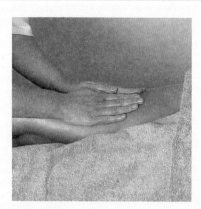

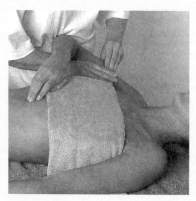

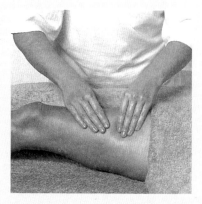

Effleurage
After applying oil, begin any massage sequence with effleurage (French for "light touching") to help the person relax and become accustomed to your hands. This is a slow and rhythmic stroking with more pressure toward the heart to increase blood and lymph flow. Keep the fingers close together and turn the fingertips slightly up.

Petrissage
Also named from French, this is a kind of kneading applied where muscle is knotted or tense and the bone is close to the surface. Work with the balls of the thumbs or fingers in steady, small circles, trapping the skin rather than sliding over it. This releases tension and stimulates blood flow through deeper arteries and veins.

Kneading
Kneading itself is for large areas where there is no bone immediately below the soft tissue. Keeping the fingers straight, pick up the flesh in one hand and pass it over to the other hand, before grasping another handful, as if you were kneading bread. This is the key technique to aid body functioning and well-being.

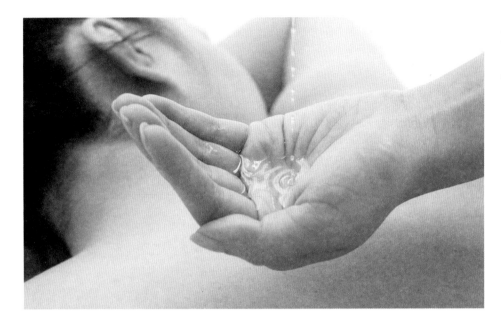

Aromatic oil, warmed in your hands, enhances a massage.

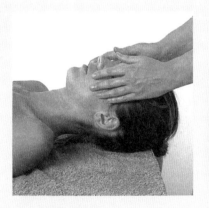

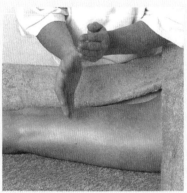

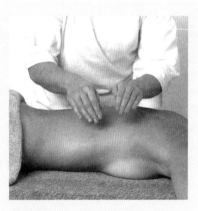

Tapotement

Meaning "tapping," this is another French-named massage technique. It is applied to small muscles, such as those of the face, to tone them. It works by contracting, then relaxing, the blood vessels, thus improving circulation. Think of lightly falling raindrops as you quickly and freely tap loose fingertips over the face, avoiding the eyes.

Hacking

This has a similar tonic effect, but is applied to larger muscles, such as those in the back, shoulders, and thighs. Hold fingers together and use the little finger edges of each hand in turn. Relax the hands slightly to avoid causing pain. Keeping the wrists loose, hack by bringing each hand up and down quickly in a chopping motion. Practice on your thigh first.

Cupping

This is done with hands bent where the fingers join the palms. The fingers and thumbs should be kept close together to create a mini-vacuum. Quickly raise and lower your cupped hands on the sides of the back, shoulders, and thighs to produce a sound like trotting hooves. This draws blood to the surface to revive the skin and reinvigorate the muscle tissue.

BREATHING THERAPY

We tend not to think much about our breathing, since it is such an automatic process, but how we breathe can have a significant effect on our health. The word "respiration" contains the root of the word "spirit," and some cultures consider the breath as sacred. Similarly, the word "inspiration," which medically means breathing in, is considered by many to be the equivalent of a divine spark.

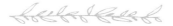

Breathing in contracts the diaphragm attached to the bottom ribs, helping the lungs to fill with air; as the diaphragm relaxes on the out-breath, carbon dioxide is exhaled.

Physically, breathing is initiated by the muscles of the diaphragm and those between the ribs contracting and relaxing. As they contract they enlarge the lung space, causing air to rush in. When it reaches the lungs' tiny air sacs, oxygen is transferred across a membrane into the bloodstream, where it is picked up by the red blood cells and incorporated into the hemoglobin molecule to be transported by the blood to all the tissues of the body. At the same time, carbon dioxide is transferred in the opposite direction, to be exhaled by the lungs as the muscles relax.

Breathing is linked to our emotional system. When we are excited or afraid, we breathe more rapidly; when we are calm, so is our breathing. It is affected by our posture, as demonstrated by the trained singer who learns to stand or sit in a certain way so as to get the deepest breath with the least effort and produce the purest sound. The discipline of yoga emphasizes the importance of the breath as a vital link connecting body, mind, spirit, and emotions. These are some of the reasons to learn to breathe properly, rather than engaging in the unconscious breathing that most people do.

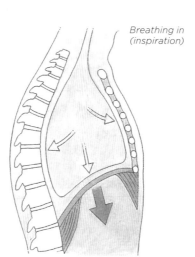

Breathing in (inspiration)

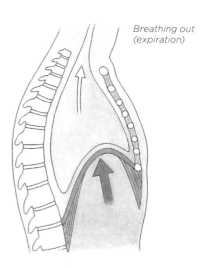

Breathing out (expiration)

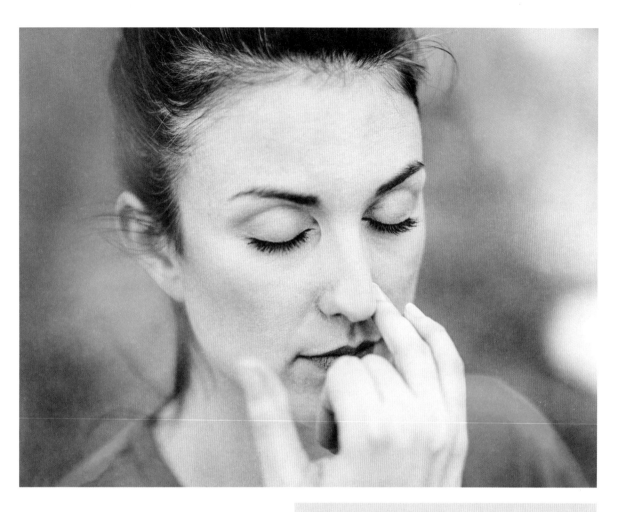

Breathing Exercise

This yoga technique improves breathing. Close the right nostril with the right thumb, bend the first and second fingers, and place the third finger by the left nostril. Breathe in to a count of four. Close the left nostril with the third finger and hold the breath for a count of 16.

Take the thumb from the right nostril and breathe slowly out to a count of eight. Then reverse the process—in through the right nostril, hold, and out through the left. Repeat about four times at first and build up to 12.

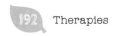

EYESIGHT TRAINING (BATES METHOD)

The Bates method was developed by Dr. W. H. Bates, a New York ophthalmologist, in the early 20th century, simply to teach people to use their eyes in a relaxed and easy manner. He had discovered that many of his patients, though responding to conventional treatment, were still complaining of headaches and eyestrain.

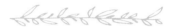

We see by means of light waves that enter the eye through the iris and are focused on the retina by the lens. Retinal cells form them into an upside-down and reversed image that travels through the blind spot via the optic nerve to the brain, where it is righted.

Vision is pure sensation. Images are presented directly to the brain for interpretation without the intervention of the intellect. What determines the accuracy of that interpretation is the attention we pay to what we are looking at. Attention must flow outward, embracing the object without distraction. It must not be forced, but must flow naturally instead. It is a matter of being mentally quiet and letting sight come. This concept is at the heart of the Bates method.

The most important "technique" that the Bates method teaches is to blink your eyes more often than you perhaps think is necessary. This is nature's way of lubricating the eyeball and breaks up the act of staring, which tires the eye muscles. Other "pearls" from the Bates method to help you relax your eyes while strengthening your eyesight are palming, splashing, and changing focus. Practice them without glasses or contact lenses and do them every day to achieve maximum benefit.

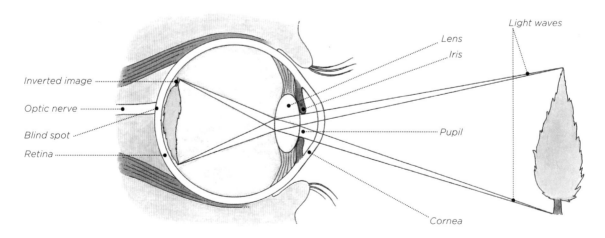

Light waves

Lens

Iris

Inverted image

Optic nerve

Blind spot

Retina

Pupil

Cornea

THE STRUCTURE OF THE EYE AND HOW WE SEE

Bates Exercises

"Palm" your eyes

This is second only to blinking as an aid to relaxed vision. Rest your elbows on a table and then cover your closed eyes with your palms, cupping your hands so that they do not touch the eyelids. Think about a pleasant place or experience. Continue in this way for about 10 minutes and repeat several times a day.

Splash your eyes

Splash your closed eyes alternately with hot and cold water. Do it on arising, with first hot and then cold water, and again before retiring, this time with first cold and then hot water. This stimulates circulation around the eyes and relieves congestion.

Change focus

Change the focus of the eyes from far to near and back to far again. This relieves the strain of focusing on one distance for a long time. You can do this while you are driving without disturbing your attention to the road. You will find that your eyes will be much less tired after a long journey.

Sunning drill

The Bates method also recommends a "sunning drill" that involves facing the sun with your eyes closed and allowing the sun to warm each cheek for two minutes.

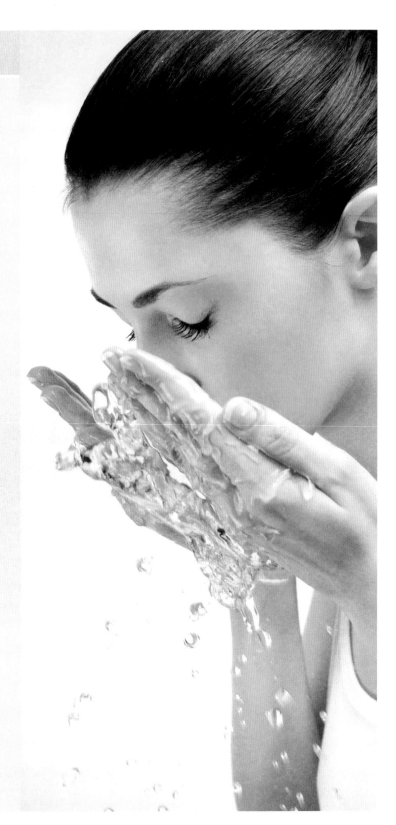

THERAPIES RELATING TO OUR VITAL ENERGY

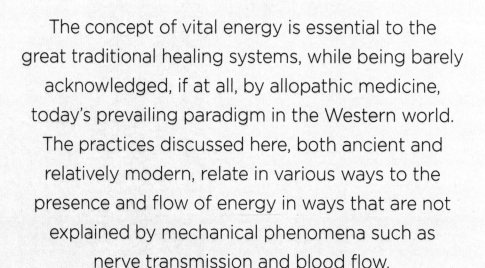

The concept of vital energy is essential to the great traditional healing systems, while being barely acknowledged, if at all, by allopathic medicine, today's prevailing paradigm in the Western world. The practices discussed here, both ancient and relatively modern, relate in various ways to the presence and flow of energy in ways that are not explained by mechanical phenomena such as nerve transmission and blood flow.

REFLEXOLOGY

Reflexology is an ancient therapy designed to bring the body back into balance after it has lost its center in the course of harmful living practices. The origin of the practice is obscure—it may have come from China. The practice has been re-energized in recent years and taught extensively in Europe and America, first by Dr. William Fitzgerald and then by Eunice Bingham, who was instrumental in mapping out the reflex areas of the feet.

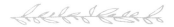

The basic premise is that our internal organs have corresponding reflex points at the body surface. The most sensitive and easily accessible areas are the feet, the hands, and the external parts of the ears. The feet are by far the most commonly used area. The principles of reflexology have been most thoroughly studied in reference to the feet, and practitioners find foot massage highly acceptable to their clients.

Reflexology has the advantage of being easily learned and beneficially practiced by a lay person who is willing to make a study of the technique. It is described in careful and understandable language in several good books. As with any hands-on technique, one's ability and sensitivity will be enhanced by learning from an experienced practitioner and by repeated use of the technique, which can easily and safely be done with friends or family members who are bound to respond to its soothing effects.

Reflexology is well-suited to home practice, because it is not difficult to create an ambience that is pleasant and comfortable and that will give the greatest benefit for both the giver and the receiver. It is important for the one whose feet are being treated to be really relaxed and comfortable. A recliner with a slightly raised footrest is ideal, but lacking this, an armchair will serve the purpose.

The recipient should be wearing comfortable, loose-fitting clothes with legs bare to the knees. It is useful to have a fuzzy towel handy in which to drape the leg and foot not being worked upon. The practitioner can sit

A good reflexologist will attempt to attune themselves to the person they are treating as well as manipulate the feet.

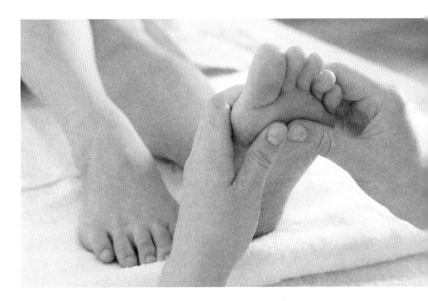

in a chair or on a stool within relaxed, easy reach of the subject's feet. Some reflexologists prefer to use no talc or lotion in their massage; others use a little, especially on dry or rough skin. Soft music is sometimes helpful in creating a pleasant atmosphere and may help the receiver to feel no need to talk, thereby encouraging a deeper level of comfort.

The actual details of how to touch, press, and manipulate the feet need to be learned from reading, private demonstration, or by attending a workshop. Once a technique is seen and understood, the giver may want to vary the procedure, always sensitive to the comfort level of the recipient. It is desirable to start with a gentle, flowing exploration of the feet and lower legs, giving the recipient a feeling of being welcome and accepted. It also serves to establish a connection on both physical and spiritual levels.

There should be no sense of a time crunch. "There is no time in the forest" is a good thought to hold. When the session is completed, the receiver should be warm, cozy, and peaceful.

Reflexology is a delightful sharing experience for couples, friends, all children, and elderly people, who need to receive special care.

A variation of reflexology, called metamorphic therapy, which was intuited by an English reflexologist named Robert St. John, is a quite astonishing reflex system in the feet. It is related not to the areas of the body but to the sequence of time of gestation in the womb. As reflexology releases stresses in the organs, metamorphic therapy (first called prenatal therapy) deals with patterns of stress that were set up in the 38 weeks of gestation. The therapy is simple, but must be practiced in a centered way. It consists of manipulation of the spinal reflexes in the feet, from the big toe through the arch to the heel. St. John's theory was that the stages of developing consciousness could be blocked during gestation, by such things as shock, emotional trauma, illness, or drugs, causing the child to become "stuck in time."

While the greatest benefits of reflexology come from treating or being treated by another experienced person, you can gain useful experience with certain techniques—such as keeping up a constant, even pressure and a steady rhythm. Manipulating the appropriate reflex points will also help to relieve your own symptoms and increase your well-being.

Reflexology Points

Reflexology works on the principle that energy zones within the body can be stimulated through the feet, where reflex areas correspond to different parts of the body. Massage techniques applied to the appropriate area seek to clear tension and remove impurities, encouraging body and mind to function harmoniously and healing to take place. The points shown below represent those referred to in the Symptoms section. You will learn about many more points if you choose to pursue this therapy further with a teacher. Note that the points are the same on both feet except where indicated; some have been shown on one foot only for clarity.

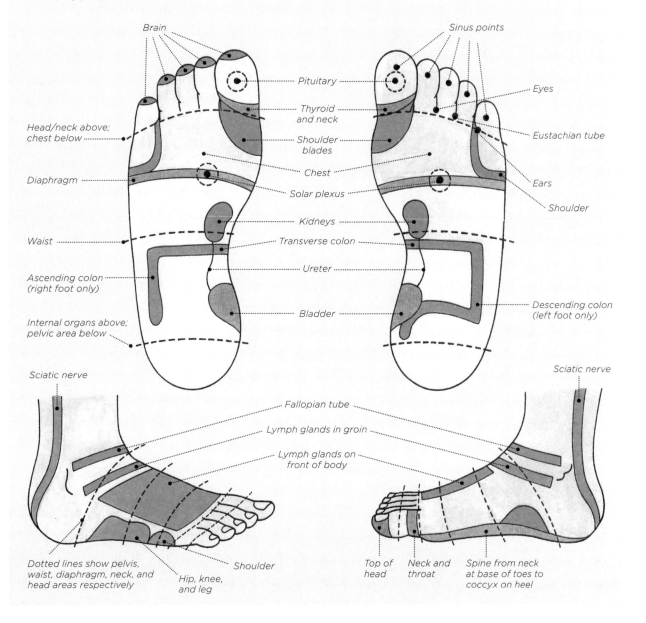

Brain

Sinus points

Pituitary

Eyes

Thyroid and neck

Head/neck above; chest below

Shoulder blades

Eustachian tube

Diaphragm

Chest

Solar plexus

Ears

Shoulder

Kidneys

Waist

Transverse colon

Ascending colon (right foot only)

Ureter

Descending colon (left foot only)

Internal organs above; pelvic area below

Bladder

Sciatic nerve

Sciatic nerve

Fallopian tube

Lymph glands in groin

Lymph glands on front of body

Dotted lines show pelvis, waist, diaphragm, neck, and head areas respectively

Shoulder

Hip, knee, and leg

Top of head

Neck and throat

Spine from neck at base of toes to coccyx on heel

Basic Reflexology Sequence

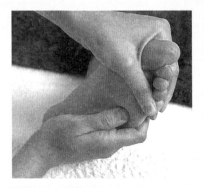

Applying pressure
Slightly bend the thumb to avoid flexing it backward when applying pressure—here to the shoulder blade point. Support with the other hand and linger with gentle, constant pressure.

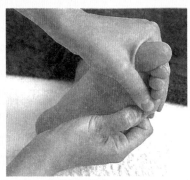

Thumb-walking
Bend the joint nearest the nail but keep the lower one comfortably straight. Each time the thumb bends, a tiny sliding step forward is taken, helped by talc on the skin.

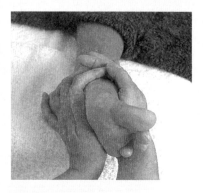

Stroking
Punctuate the working of reflex points with relaxing stroking. With one hand cupping the foot underneath and the other on top, slowly slide up from toes to ankle. Circle back down and repeat.

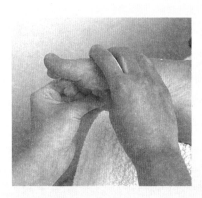

Scrunching
Scrunch as an opening movement, after applying talc, to free the foot of muscular tension. Twist each hand in opposite directions, working from just under the toes to the ankle.

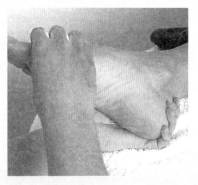

Rotating ankle I
To release tension from the ankle at the start of a reflexology treatment, cup the heel in one relaxed hand while the other, lightly holding the chest area, slowly rotates the foot.

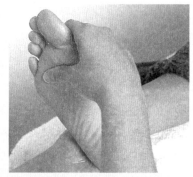

Rotating ankle II
Rotate the ankle slowly one way, then the other. You may need to make smaller movements or change direction at varying intervals if the person tries to join in. Stop if they cannot relax.

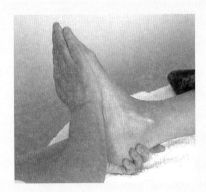

Pushing

This can help the foot, leg, and lower back. Cradle the heel in one hand while pressing forward with the other on the ball of the foot. Draw the heel back at the same time, without forcing.

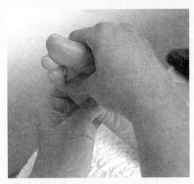

Rotating solar plexus

With one thumb on the solar plexus point (at diaphragm level between the second and third toes), rotate the foot above with a gentle, relaxing rhythm—better than ankle rotation for some.

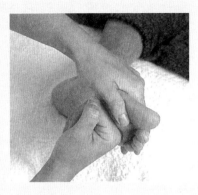

Circular caress

To comfort, make a fist with one hand and press the back of the fingers (not the knuckles) into the ball of the foot. Slowly, firmly rotate the fist. Use the heel of the hand in times of anxiety.

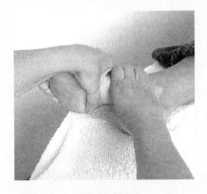

Spinal scrunch/twist

To ease the spinal reflex after thumb-walking, rest both hands on top of the foot, with thumbs together underneath. Move the hand nearest the toes back and forth to twist the reflex gently.

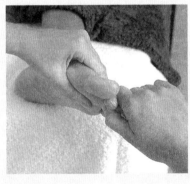

Pulling toes

Relax the neck to finish by holding each toe in turn, with thumb pad underneath and the side of the index finger above. Smoothly ease each toe toward you.

"Some evidence of reflexology's relaxing qualities is the fact that many people feel like sleeping after a treatment."

ACUPRESSURE

Acupressure is an aspect of acupuncture, which in turn is just one element of Oriental medicine. Acupressure can be used with benefit at home; acupuncture, which requires the services of a highly trained practitioner, cannot.

Acupressure started over 4,500 years ago and is still used for the treatment of ailments today.

Acupressure is an easily learned technique that can access certain of the acupuncture points, with similar beneficial results. A great many of the points can be reached with one's own hands; a friend can help with the more inaccessible ones. The practice of Shiatsu—the Japanese word for finger (shi) pressure (atsu)—is the Japanese equivalent of acupressure and is based on the same principles as acupuncture.

Traditional Oriental medicine has ancient roots. It contains much wisdom about life. Acupuncture, diet, manipulation and massage, hydrotherapy, herbal therapy, sun and air therapy, and exercise are among its complex manifestations. Writings on acupuncture go back 4,500 years, to the publication of the first books of the Nei Ching, which took approximately 1,500 years to complete.

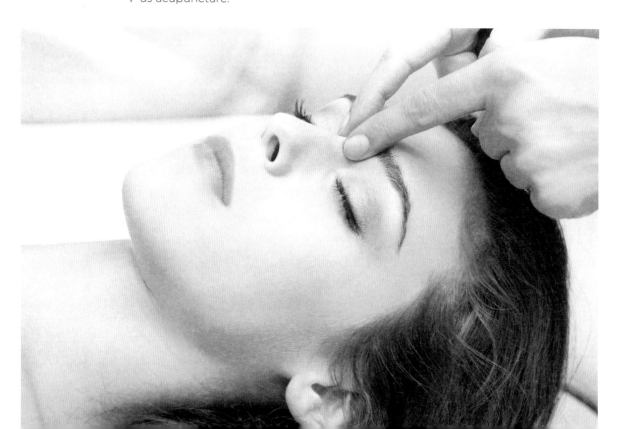

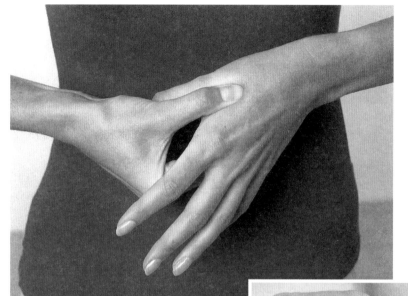

Large intestine 4 is known as the "Great Eliminator." It is one of the most useful and accessible acupressure points and is located in the triangle at the base of the thumb and forefinger. Treat a headache by rotating your thumb firmly on the point—but not when pregnant.

ACUPUNCTURE

Acupuncture is based on the theory that there are in the body two complementary energy flows called yin and yang, in an overall concept of energy known as chi or life force. Yin and yang are expressed as day and night, male and female, hot and cold, life and death—everything in the universe. Every aspect has an opposing one that is at the same time complementary. Health is dependent on the balance of yin and yang, both within the body and within the whole universe. These energy flows circulate in the body along meridians, or circuits, that can be measured by electronic and other means. There are 26 main meridians, each representing a different body function or organ. Along these meridians are at least 800 points known as acupuncture points, which have been found to affect the energy flow when acupuncture needles are placed on them. When the flow is altered appropriately, the balance within that circuit, and thus the health of that system, is restored. Acupuncture anesthesia is notably successful for surgery of the upper part of the body.

Symptoms that are known to have been successfully treated include migraine, tension headache, ulcers and digestive problems, back pain, arthritis, fibromyalgia, neuritis, rheumatism, dermatitis, eczema, psoriasis, and other skin conditions, high blood pressure, anxiety, depression, asthma, bronchitis, and many others.

Pressure points such as the "Great Eliminator" are stimulated in both acupressure and acupuncture.

Acupressure Points

Acupressure stimulates the flow of energy, or chi, circulating along meridians throughout the body that are linked to different organs. Applying pressure to the key points on the meridians works like acupuncture to treat symptoms and restore a healthy balance to the corresponding area. The points shown below represent those referred to in the Symptoms section. You will learn about many more acupressure points if you choose to pursue this therapy further with a teacher.

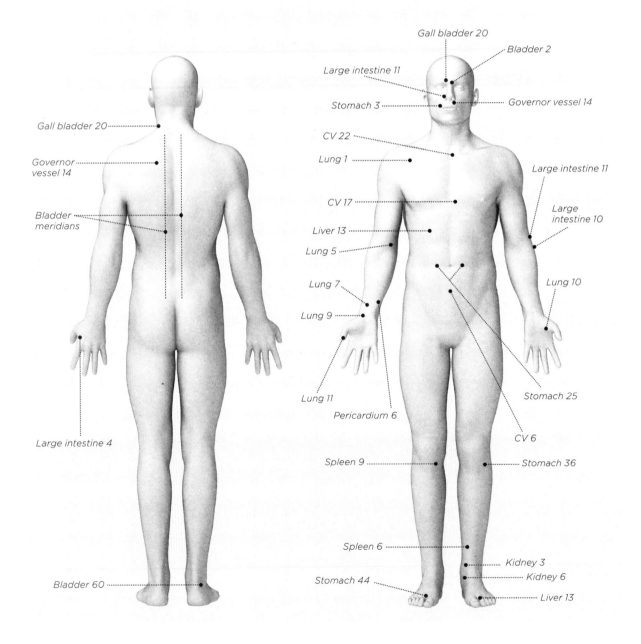

Gall bladder 20

Bladder 2

Large intestine 11

Governor vessel 14

Stomach 3

CV 22

Lung 1

Large intestine 11

CV 17

Large intestine 10

Liver 13

Lung 5

Lung 7

Lung 10

Lung 9

Lung 11

Stomach 25

Pericardium 6

CV 6

Spleen 9

Stomach 36

Spleen 6

Kidney 3

Stomach 44

Kidney 6

Liver 13

Gall bladder 20

Governor vessel 14

Bladder meridians

Large intestine 4

Bladder 60

Basic Acupressure Sequence

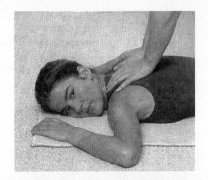

Getting into position

Before applying pressure to any points, practice crawling like a baby to feel centered in your hara—the powerful core of the body's energy, situated about two fingers ' width below the navel. As you begin treatment, keep your weight central to the person being treated, with your back easy and your hands and wrists relaxed. Place your hands at the top of the back, one at each shoulder.

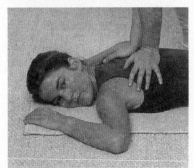

Releasing muscular tension

Using gravity and your body weight only (not physical force), "walk " your hands down the sides of the spine. This should feel like a slow, heavy cat pawing down the back and releasing muscular tension. To keep your arms vertical, so that your body weight is over your hands, you will need to move your legs down your partner's body as you walk down the back.

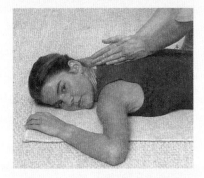

Preparing the meridian

With your own body still centered, but without any weight on your hands, "scissor" with the outside edges of your hands down the bladder meridians on either side of the spinal column. Your hands will be about 2in (5cm) apart as you slide them up and down along the spine, but gradually working down to the hips. This prepares the meridian for the stimulation to follow.

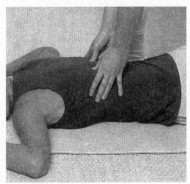

Stimulating pressure points

Place your thumbs at the top of the energy lines just prepared. Allow your weight to let your thumbs sink into two points on either side of the spinal column. Allow increased pressure as you both breathe out; relieve the weight as you inhale or if there is discomfort. On an in-breath, slide down the bladder meridians to work the next point, and so on down to the coccyx.

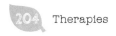

YOGA

Yoga is a philosophy embracing every aspect of life—spiritual, mental, emotional, and physical. It is a system of self-improvement, or conscious evolution, that has itself evolved and modified over the 6,000 years of its known existence.

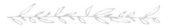

Hatha yoga is the physical aspect of yoga practice, but this only makes up a small section of yoga as a whole.

Yoga came to the West from India a century or so ago, via returning soldiers and civil servants. There are a number of classic writings expounding the principles and concepts of yoga, of which the greatest is the Bhagavad Gita, written about 300 A.D., which presents in detail the five main systems of yoga.

- Gnana yoga: the spiritual aspect
- Bhakti yoga: the emotional aspect
- Raja yoga: the mental aspect
- Karma yoga: the yoga of social responsibility
- Hatha yoga: the physical aspect (in its rudimentary form)

It is through the latter, hatha yoga, that most Westerners are introduced to the philosophy. Many people believe that this is yoga and are largely ignorant of the totality of yoga as a great philosophy of life. Hatha yoga was actually the most recent aspect to be fully developed (c. 1500 A.D.).

A typical hatha yoga class consists of the following.

- Exercises are performed standing, kneeling, lying on the back and the front, and inverted. For every posture (asana), there is a counter-posture.
- Kriyas, techniques that cleanse all parts of the alimentary tract, are learned.
- Techniques for deep relaxation are learned.
- Breathing exercises (pranayama) are performed.
- Meditaton is practiced.
- Short talks are given dealing with various aspects of yoga, philosophy, practice, correct posture, diet, or emotional issues. Occasional discussions may ensue on the subjects of the other yogas noted above, on siddha, the yoga of psychic powers, on reincarnation, or on karma, the law of cause and effect.

Self-help and self-education are the rule in yoga therapy. Only changes generated from within are considered to be of real value in personal development. Yoga students learn to come to a high state of awareness, to feel their way into their bodies, minds, emotions, and value judgments, and to question their ways of dealing with their environment and personal relationships. The yoga teacher acts as a guide to assist in this internal awakening.

"Yoga promotes not only physical mobility but a positive mental and emotional approach that can have profound psychological benefits."

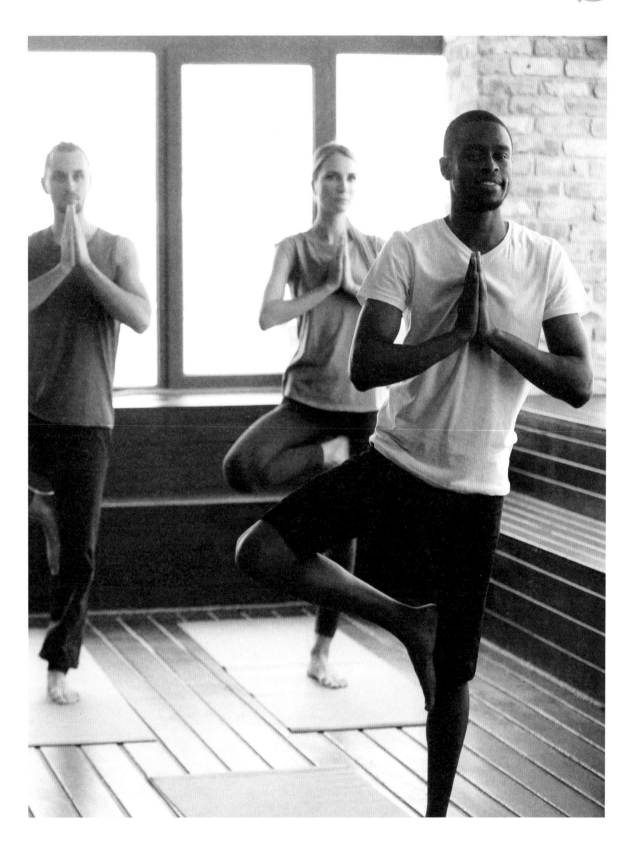

Basic Yoga Postures

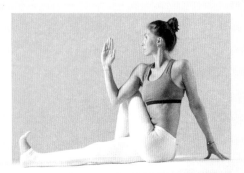

Spinal twist

Sit upright with your legs out, feet together and toes up. Bend the left leg, bringing it over the right leg at the knee joint. Then bring the right arm against the left knee. Breathe in.

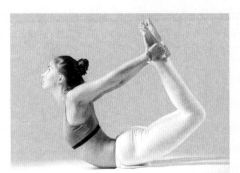

Bow

Lie face down, feet together. Breathe in. As you breathe out, lift head, shoulders, and chest, bend the knees, and bring feet toward the head. Hold the out-breath and then come gently down.

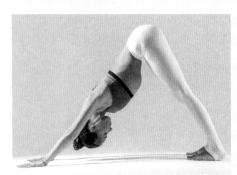

Dog

Drop onto all fours, knees apart and palms forward. Practice lowering and arching the back on in- and out-breaths. Straighten the legs on an out-breath, thrusting the buttocks into the air.

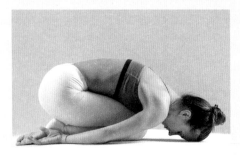

Cat

Sink back onto the heels, with hands beside the feet, palms facing upward and forehead touching the ground. Remain relaxed like this for two or three minutes before getting up slowly.

Half shoulder stand

Lie on your back, legs together, and raise legs and trunk as you breathe in. When the legs reach a vertical position, lightly hold the small of the back. Hold the position, breathing slowly.

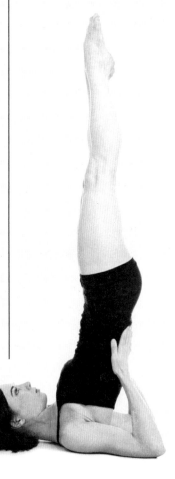

Basic Yoga Sequence—"Salute to the Sun"

The "Salute to the Sun" sequence is ideal for boosting energy levels—particularly if performed on rising—and for improving posture and flexibility.

1 Stand upright, knees and feet together. Hold palms together close to chest, with fingers up.

2 Breathing in, step to the right, raise arms over head, palms up, reaching backward.

3 Breathe out and lean forward without bending knees, reaching down as far as you can.

4 Breathe in. Bend knees, take left leg back, resting knee on floor. Raise arms, palms together.

5 Holding your breath, extend both legs and raise body on straight arms, palms flat.

6 Drop to knees, keeping toes tucked under and gaze straight ahead. Stay as still as possible.

7 Breathing out, sit back on heels, with feet still raised on toes. Stretch arms forward.

8 Breathe in and dive gently forward, bending elbows and sliding chin close to floor.

9 Still breathing in, straighten arms and swing hips forward, curving spine and looking up.

10 Breathe out, raise hips, and drop toes and heels flat onto the floor, keeping legs straight.

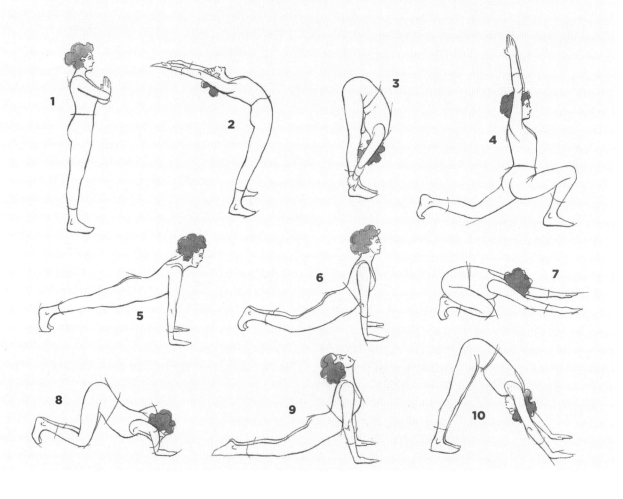

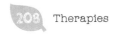

TAI CHI

Tai chi has been called "meditation in motion." Its origins are lost in antiquity, though its roots come from Chinese martial arts training. In the West it is known entirely for its health, exercise, and spiritual aspects.

Tai chi is based on intrinsic energy, and uses the same invisible channels as acupuncture.

Tai chi is all about balance—an important element of Chinese culture.

Its modern applications developed in 19th-century China. Of the five styles that are best known today—Chen, Yang, Wu, Sun, and Hao—the Yang style is the most widely taught. In the 1950s, leading Chinese tai chi experts laid down a number of forms or movement sequences that have been gaining in popularity ever since. These forms consist of postures connected in such a way that a continuous chain of movement occurs. The form teaches movement as an event in which the whole body participates, not just isolated muscle groups.

The basic concept on which tai chi is based is chi, or intrinsic energy. In the theory of tai chi, the chi flows downward through invisible channels to all parts of the body. These are the same channels, or meridians, that are basic to acupuncture, and indeed to all of traditional Chinese medicine. The chi energy helps all the organs and fluids of the body to function properly. When one of the channels becomes blocked, the chi cannot flow as it should; when a channel is too open, the chi flows too freely.

In intelligent people there is an excess of energy and activity (hence chi) in the upper part of the body, the activity being fiery and agitated. The lower part of the body is calmer, like still water. Tai chi aims to bring the fire down into the lower part and the water into the upper part until the proper balance exists. This is done through learning first the proper alignment of the parts of the body, then by learning a number of forms that apply in different situations. Another idea that is basic to tai chi is that the mind (yi) leads the chi, which suggests that we should in all things be mindful of what we do from moment to moment.

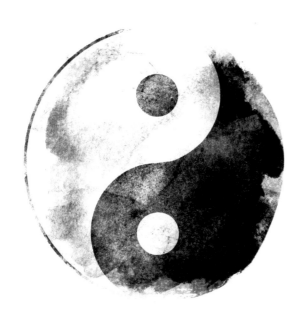

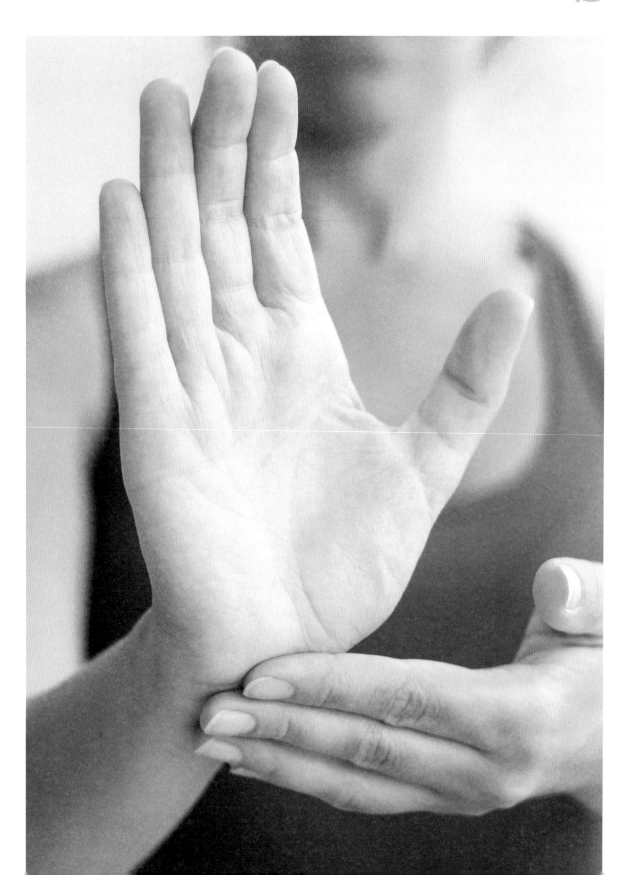

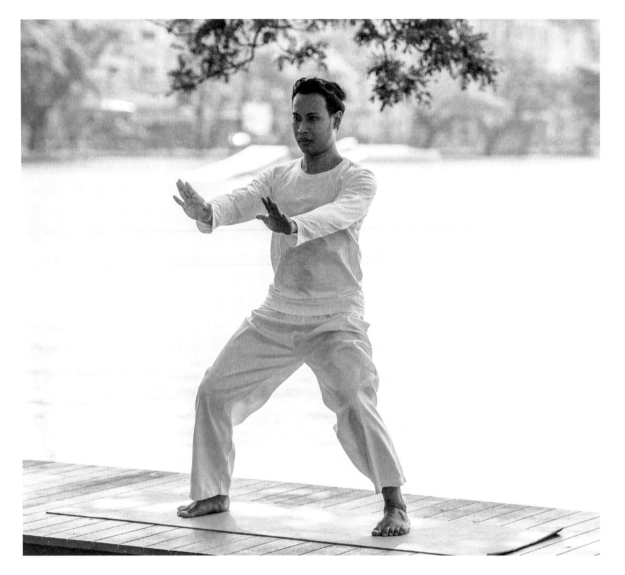

The Chinese traditionally practice tai chi movements in the open air.

The specific benefits of tai chi include the following.

- It improves the relationship of the head to the neck and spine, thus reducing strain on muscles that maintain posture.
- It improves the circulation of energy and chi.
- It achieves balance in the tone of the muscles and teaches the correct use of the joints.
- It teaches uniform body relaxation and energy distribution, which promotes better digestion.
- It helps to reduce stress.

The success of tai chi depends on learning its techniques properly and then on integrating the practice into one's everyday life. Much can be learned by reading, but time with a qualified teacher will be time well spent, as small differences in technique can be critical.

Basic Tai Chi Sequence—"Brush Knee and Push"

1 Turn left foot in. Lower right palm, raise left palm. Look over right shoulder.

2 Right foot out. Lower, then raise right palm, circling left palm down across chest.

3 Shift weight to right leg. Swivel to East, left heel up, right hand rising to ear.

4 Step East, turning body; left palm above left knee, right hand pushing forward.

5 Raise left toes. Turn waist left. Raise left palm, point right fingers at left elbow.

6 Step right foot, heel up; right hand "brushes" waist, left palm pushes forward.

7 Step directly East with right foot; complete "brush" across waist and push.

8 Shift weight back to left foot and turn right foot out, toes slightly raised.

9 Step up left foot, heel raised, close to right; repeat "brush" and push.

10 Shift weight back to left and turn right foot out, toes slightly raised.

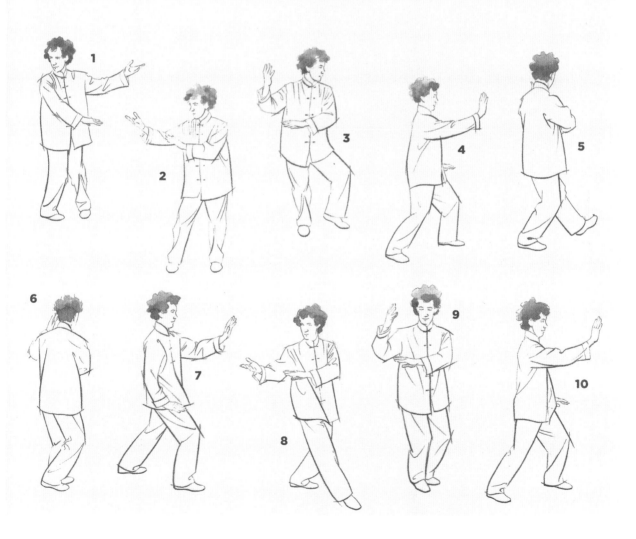

THERAPEUTIC TOUCH

Therapeutic touch is a hands-on healing technique developed and tested by Dr. Dolores Krieger, an R.N. and nursing professor at New York University in the early 1970s. In carefully constructed experiments, Krieger was able to demonstrate the beneficial effect that a caring person can have on an ill person by means of touch.

The practical importance of this is to reinforce the fact that careful and loving attention to a sick person in the home will have a very beneficial effect on that person. A simple back massage with gentle aromatic oil, a foot massage, or even putting on soothing or favorite music, when done lovingly and attentively, will elevate the spirits of the sick person, reduce pain, and induce relaxation. The only prerequisites needed to perform such a service are gentle, willing hands and a loving heart.

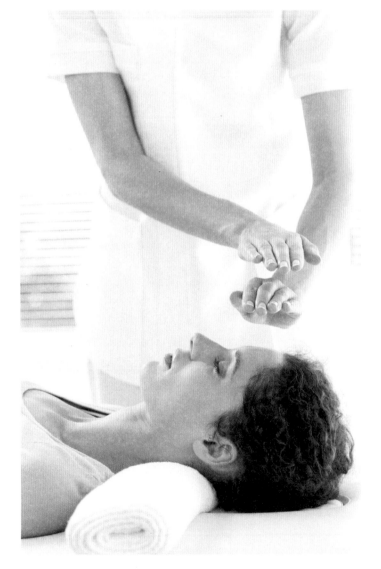

Touch and physical closeness can be used in many ways to ease pain. The spiritual healer aims to transmit power through a "laying on of hands," usually on or above the head.

APPLIED KINESIOLOGY

Applied kinesiology is the name given to a system of muscle testing. Certain muscle groups have been found to be related to the major internal systems of the body, in that they reflect imbalances in those systems. By testing muscular strength, the practitioner assesses the state of the relevant internal system (e.g. gastrointestinal).

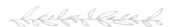

By then placing on the tongue a sample of food or a nutritional supplement known to be helpful, a previously weak-testing muscle can be seen to convert to a strong-testing one. In the hands of a trained practitioner, this method becomes quite sophisticated, but the average person can learn to develop the technique to a surprisingly high level. This may be useful in determining, for example, whether a food is causing a harmful reaction in the body due to allergy or hypersensitivity, and also in problems of an emotional or behavioral nature.

To become proficient in this method, it is essential to learn from an experienced and qualified instructor. The changes in muscle reaction are definite but subtle. Personal instruction is needed to develop the ability to detect such muscle changes. You cannot carry out this technique alone at home, as you need both a tester and a subject.

A kinesiologist tests for food allergy by assessing muscle strength.

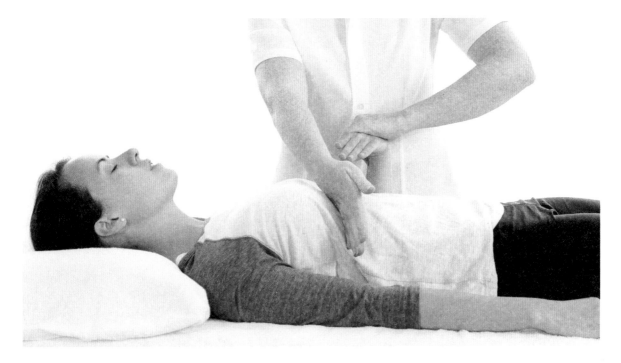

THERAPIES RELATING TO THE MIND, EMOTIONS, AND SPIRIT

This diverse group of therapies have to do with the nonphysical aspects of our being. They include considerations of the interaction of the invisible mind with the physical body, about which so much has been written; our emotional reactions, which have mostly to do with our interactions with others; and our spiritual life, that ineffable and all-pervasive realm, supremely important and very difficult for the mind to comprehend.

MEDITATION

Meditation is an ancient art, as old as recorded history. It is an integral part of the East Indian tradition that goes back thousands of years. It has also been a part of the fabric of other cultures around the world, in some instances for many centuries. Yet despite its antiquity, it is the subject of intense interest, study, and practice in the 21st century.

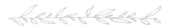

Swami Rama, the renowned Indian teacher, has said that "meditation is the state of being established in one's own essential nature." The simplicity of this statement seems to bear witness to its truth and gives sufficient reason to consider adopting the practice. It is so important to come to know who we truly are and to separate for ourselves our "essential nature" from the images of ourselves that we present to the outside world. If we fail to do this, we run a serious risk of coming to believe that the image is the real person. Many people build their lives on this kind of incorrect conclusion, leading to untold conflict within themselves. The truth about who we are lies deep within us, and we need to discover a reliable and repeatable path to that center of serenity and truth.

Meditation is not something apart from our daily lives; if we pursue it, we find that the whole of living can become a meditation. This should be our aim in meditation—to refine our consciousness so that every thought and action are in tune with the universal plan and, therefore, sacred. This may sound quite grand, but it is within the reach of anyone who desires it. In order to be healthy and whole, we must be in harmony within ourselves, and at the same time in harmony with other beings and with universal purposes. It is disharmony in these areas that leaves us fragmented and confused as to the meaning and direction of our lives, and paves the way for a multitude of physical illnesses that can afflict us.

There is an unbreakable bond in each of us that unites body, mind, emotions, and spirit. This is not something we must achieve—it is an immutable fact of our nature. Meditation is capable of opening existing bridges between various aspects of our nature. There is no need to build the bridges—they are already there! They just need to be swept off, scraped, and painted, so to speak, and they will be ready to use.

The Sanskrit symbol for the "sacred sound" OM, which is used widely in meditation to clear and focus the mind.

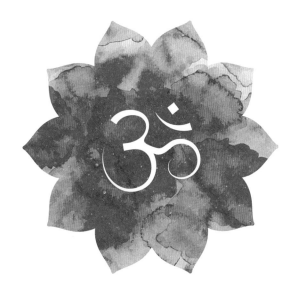

Meditation can bring us to the calm center of our essential nature, uniting body, mind, emotions, and spirit.

Similarly, bridges exist between us and all the other beings and conditions in the universe, because we are all parts of the same cosmic idea. Once they are properly tended, the right interactions among all beings can be expected to take place. In this manner, the tensions we experience within ourselves and with those outside ourselves will gradually ease. But continual maintenance of our precious bridges must be carried out if they are to give us uninterrupted service. That is the function that can be served by making our lives an unending meditation.

Many studies have been done by medical investigators regarding the effects of meditation on physiological processes. Such studies repeatedly show beneficial effects on blood pressure, heart rate and rhythm, digestive patterns, nerve conduction, muscle function, and many other parameters. It is a happy circumstance that people's subjective appraisal has largely been supported by reliable medical studies.

The next question is: How shall I meditate and what will it be like? The answer to the second part of the question is that it will be different for you than it is or has been for anyone else! It has been said that there are as many different kinds of meditation as there are people who meditate. You are already meditating from time to time, as you sit before the fire, becoming absorbed in watching the dancing flames, or when you are lured into the comfortable chair next to the audio player by the strains of a beautiful work of music. You know you have been meditating when you look up at the clock and note that a chunk of time has passed without your realizing it! Just that little spell of meditation has been extremely good for you. But it was what we might call accidental; what is wanted now is meditation that is intentional—and regular. It will be deep and exquisite and refreshing to the soul.

How then do you begin? Only a few things are required.

- You need a regular time of day that can safely be set aside. Try getting up a half hour earlier than usual.
- You need a special place in your home that is quiet, a little remote perhaps, and has a good feeling.
- You need a chair or a cushion that feels good to you. Sit upright—you do not want to fall asleep.
- You should wear loose-fitting, comfortable clothes.

Now that you are comfortably settled, close your eyes, relax your muscles, let go of all thoughts, and be aware of your breathing. For the moment, your mental screen is blank. Thoughts will inevitably come back to you—we are so accustomed to having them! When a thought occurs, be aware of it—do not pretend it is not there—but then let go of it and go back to your breathing. You may experience colors or a pleasant remembered scene. Those can be accepted. You will find that you are transported to a different reality and that it is very restful. Eventually you will become aware that perhaps it is time to return to everyday reality. Take a few moments to adjust to this idea and then be aware of your muscles, move your shoulders, stretch a little, and slowly and gently open your eyes.

"When the mind is at rest, it has, like the body, a much greater capacity for healing itself. Meditation is a way of resting your mind beyond simply thinking nothing or daydreaming."

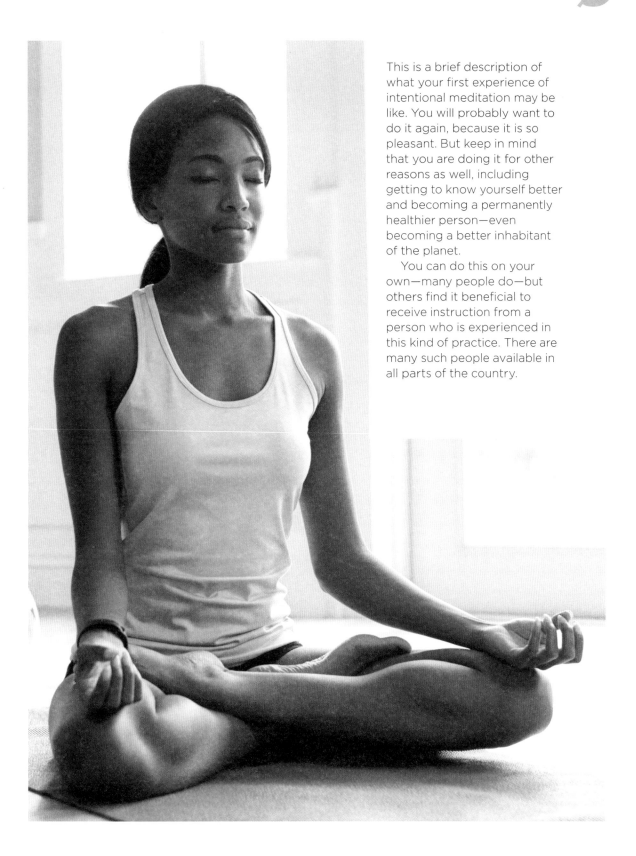

This is a brief description of what your first experience of intentional meditation may be like. You will probably want to do it again, because it is so pleasant. But keep in mind that you are doing it for other reasons as well, including getting to know yourself better and becoming a permanently healthier person—even becoming a better inhabitant of the planet.

You can do this on your own—many people do—but others find it beneficial to receive instruction from a person who is experienced in this kind of practice. There are many such people available in all parts of the country.

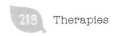

IMAGERY

Imagery is a form of human thought and is therefore universal. It is a "language" we all possess, quite apart from the cultural language that we learn at home and at school. It is the language of our dreams. Instead of words and ideas, imagery employs pictures and symbols.

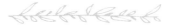

Gaining access to the personal world of images—the language of the subconscious—can help solve everyday problems as well as promote health.

It occurs spontaneously, as in dreams, which are one expression of the subconscious mind. The conscious mind speaks to us in words; the unconscious speaks in images. We have been taught to pay attention only to words, but by becoming aware of the images that are a part of our makeup, we gain access to a whole world of information that is important to us, but that we have been taught to ignore.

Guided imagery is a therapeutic technique. It is designed to help people learn the art of gaining access to their inner world of imagery, and to use that imagery for their own benefit. When someone learns to enter that realm, repeated access can be gained at will for the purpose of coming to grips with a wide variety of problems.

HYPNOSIS AND GUIDED IMAGERY

These are similar techniques, but a distinction can be made. It has been said that hypnosis is an authoritarian way to do guided imagery, while the latter is a very permissive way to do hypnosis. Guided imagery enables, while hypnosis tends to command. So it would seem that "opening oneself up to one's own imagery" is perhaps a good way of looking at what we are trying to do. Imagery has been called the navigational tool of the whole person.

There are many practical applications of imagery.

- It aids relaxation.
- It increases tolerance of acutely difficult situations.
- It provides direct relief of pain.
- It develops insight into feelings and behavior.
- It transforms troublesome patterns into more functional alternatives.
- It helps to affirm one's strengths.
- It elicits the personal meaning of an illness.
- It acts as a rehearsal for a difficult upcoming encounter.
- It affirms the positive aspects of change.
- It fosters physical healing.

As can be seen quite clearly, this list covers a broad range of issues involving personal growth as well as physical and emotional health. Imagery is uniquely suited to self-care in one's home. Its basic principles must be properly understood and must be rehearsed under the guidance of a qualified instructor to be practiced effectively. Once this is done, it is easy to carry out and be continued for as long as its use is beneficial. It is also pleasant to carry yourself into the world of images whenever you choose—it can be used as an adjunct to meditation and in other ways.

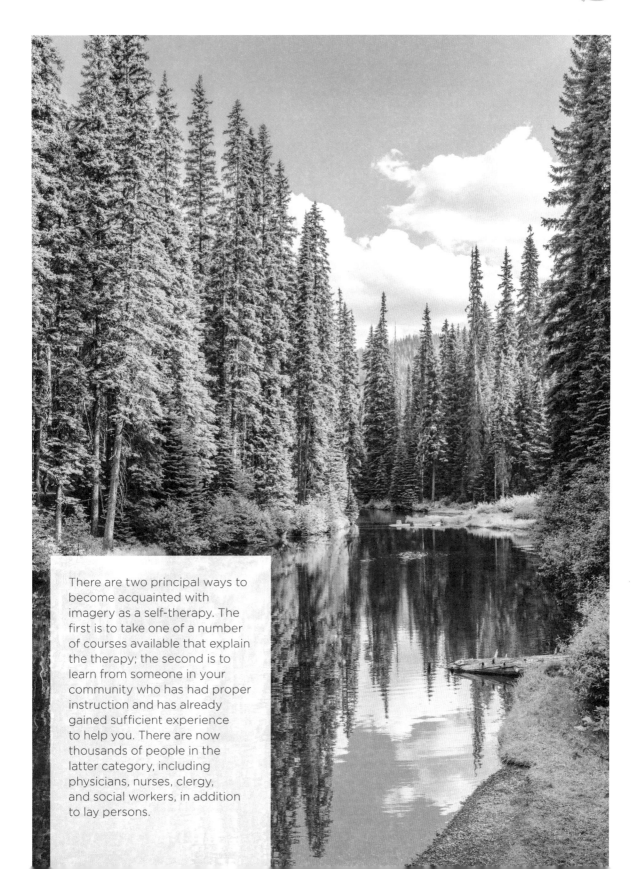

There are two principal ways to become acquainted with imagery as a self-therapy. The first is to take one of a number of courses available that explain the therapy; the second is to learn from someone in your community who has had proper instruction and has already gained sufficient experience to help you. There are now thousands of people in the latter category, including physicians, nurses, clergy, and social workers, in addition to lay persons.

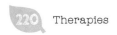

STRESS MANAGEMENT

Stress is one of the most talked about subjects in the Western world today, and well it should be. The various stresses to which we are all subjected play a major part in the erosion of our health and well-being.

One cannot talk about stress without invoking the name of Professor Hans Selye, who propounded in the early part of the 20th century the basic principles of how stress affects the human organism. Since that time, an enormous amount of study has been devoted to the subject.

Among other things, our understanding of stress has become one of the cornerstones of the field of study known as psychoneuro-immunology. This is the study of how external stresses initiate a complex chain of responses within the human organism, by way of the emotional, nervous, and immune systems. Many investigations in this field have led to new insights, paving the way to a wider use of many complementary therapies.

There are many kinds of stress that impinge upon our lives. Of all the situations and conditions that can induce stressful effects, perhaps the most significant are those involved with our relationships with other people. One of the greatest challenges we face as we embark on our life on this planet is to "learn" how best to relate to others, and conversely what ways do not work and need to be avoided. Some people seem to have a knack in relating to others, but many have great difficulty in this area, leading to problems throughout life.

The two places in which we spend virtually all of our time (after our years of schooling are finished) are the home environment and the workplace, plus shuttling back and forth from one to the other. It is clear that these must be the places where we encounter the significant people in our lives, and thus the stresses that these encounters engender.

Why are personal interactions so stressful? It would take many pages to describe all the thoughts and emotions involved, but it seems that when even two highly complex organisms (let alone 3 or 4 or 20) come into relationship, there is a tremendous potential for difficult (or pleasant) things to happen. Whatever the case, each person immediately begins "coping" with the situation and the inner systems interpret that as a challenge. Whether the interaction is pleasant or not, it is interpreted by the body as stressful.

"Relationships in the workplace are a source of stress. A first meeting with others alerts the body to challenge, whether the encounter is pleasant or not."

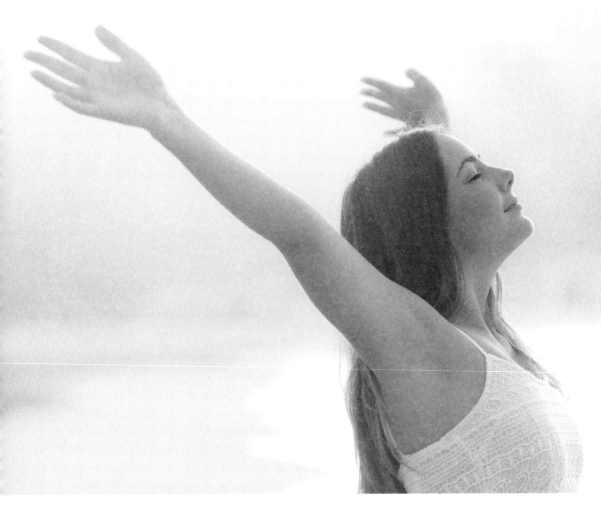

Where interactions with other people are concerned, the resulting stress is largely emotional rather than physical, mental, or spiritual. For example, upon first meeting a person, one's initial reaction might be, "I'm comfortable/uncomfortable with this person," clearly an emotional reaction, perhaps having to do with fear, attraction, or boredom.

If a person you are relating to at the moment engenders in you a negative response, an inviting option is to elect not to continue relating. The trouble comes when that person is a family member or someone you must continue to deal with at work or in some other social situation. Then you must adapt to the situation, so that you do not experience any one of a number of stress-related symptoms. Not infrequently, the person you may be having difficulty relating to is yourself, in which case it will be very important to recognize that fact, so as to make sure that someone else does not get blamed for it by mistake.

A great many therapeutic approaches have been designed to help people understand and work with various aspects of the emotional system. This is because each person is

Learning how to relax has been shown to have a powerful healing effect on both the body and mind.

Most complementary therapies, including meditation, help to reduce stress and aid relaxation.

unique, and no approach works for more than a modest percentage of people. Most approaches (except drugs, which suppress reactions) emphasize the nature of one's emotional reactions and the nature of interactions between people. Conventional therapies include psychiatry, psychology, psychotherapy, and counseling.

Beyond these, virtually every therapy described in this book has the potential to help you reduce stress in some way, by making you stronger, better balanced, more aware, or calmer. In the long run, you need to decide, after studying the choices, what direction is best for you. As you read this book thoughtfully, you will be drawn to several things that turn on a light or ring a bell for you. You may want to seek out the advice of people who are more experienced than you. In time, you will find comfort in your choices and then start to progress your ways of relating to others. When this happens, this book will have begun to serve its purpose.

GROUP THERAPY

Many of the therapies discussed in this book can be carried out individually in the home, but they can also be performed with great benefit in groups, either in group members' homes or in some central and convenient location.

The benefits of group therapy are many. Groups will often be able to secure speakers or other resource people where an individual cannot. They offer mutual support in practicing and maintaining skills, as well as moral support and encouragement. The benefits of socialization are also great.

Some therapies in some locations will only be taught to groups, with the option to carry on the practice on your own or in self-organized smaller groups. Many areas now have community bulletin boards to announce meetings of all kinds in the area. Similar bulletin boards can be accessed via computer networks. Group therapy is sometimes carried on at a fixed location, for example at a health spa, whose location is determined by a feature such as a hot spring. A great many locations are advertised now around the country in magazines focusing on health and fitness.

Another source of information is the local health food store, which usually has a magazine section as well as a bulletin board for local activities. These stores are becoming a valuable resource for those looking for organic and nutritious food, vitamins and other supplements, and information. They are proliferating as the demand for their products and services escalates.

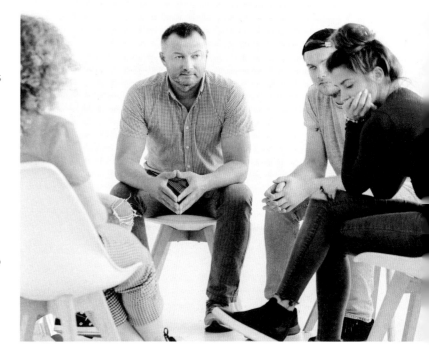

The mutual support and interest of a group can be highly beneficial, whether in talking through personal problems or learning, discussing, and practicing complementary therapies that can be continued in self-organized groups or alone at home.

MUSIC THERAPY

Music affects us as profoundly as anything we experience. Record numbers of people today say that music is a big part of their everyday life. We can hear evidence of this in music blaring from cars and see it in the jogger listening to music through earphones.

Music has charms to soothe, entrance, and touch the deepest part of our being, whether we are listeners or creators of beautiful sound.

The modern-day portability of music brings it everywhere people live, play, and work. Much of what engages so many people seems to center about the primitive beat of today's rock and pop music. Yet there is still a substantial audience for classical music, from the plainsong and chant of the Middle Ages to 21st-century atonal music. The emergence of the folk music of scores of cultures around the world, disseminated by modern technology, is another interesting musical development in our century.

All this testifies to the great effect music has on virtually all people. Different parts of the body resonate to different sounds and pitches, and, most significantly of all, certain kinds of music resound powerfully in the human spirit. It is this that gives us daily opportunity to find out what music is most able to refresh our spirit. Computer technology has made it possible to capture and re-create the world's finest music and reproduce it in the home, in the car, and on the jogging path. Those who have the gift of making music with the voice or an instrument experience an added dimension to life, but it is true that many who might make music do not do so only through lack of confidence in themselves or their abilities.

So music is really therapy for millions of people in our culture, whether they make it or merely listen to it. It reaches its greatest significance when it becomes part of the spiritual life. Here it may be combined with the most meaningful poetry the world has known, or strike deep chords within us that speak of the infinite and our part of that reality. Every significant religious tradition contains music that embodies the spirituality and the longing of the people.

There are many ways to gain access to music for healing purposes. Catalogs can be found at music stores, magazines describing healing music are often found in health food stores, and the internet, of course, is a vast resource of music and information.

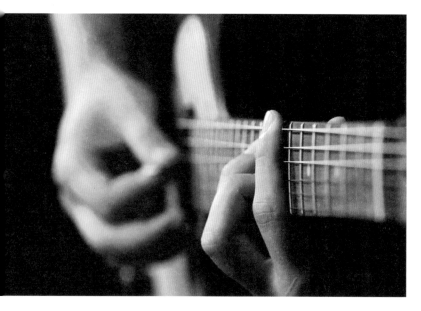

ART AND COLOR THERAPY

People have used art, light, and color to evoke certain responses since ancient times. The sanctuaries of Egyptian and Greek temples were painted in colors thought to have been chosen deliberately for their effect. Psychological as well as spiritual effects have been studied and produced in all parts of the world.

Research indicates that color is perceived not only by the eyes, but also by the skin and in dreams and meditation. The colors used in our environment have a definite effect on our moods and attitudes. A color therapist uses the colors in fabrics, wallpaper, paint, and illumination to produce desired effects. Color is also utilized through imagery, counseling, and guided meditation, with energizing, clarifying, or calming effects. Color is also an element of aura therapy, in which a therapist sensitive to the colors in people's auras can counsel them and monitor changes in the aura.

Through the medium of art therapy, both adults and children can be helped to express their inner needs and desires, and to record the content of dreams and meditations. Art can be a key to the door of the inner mind, externalizing thoughts and feelings, and thus giving insight into hidden concerns that may be preventing a person from achieving full potential in life. The following are some of the practical situations in which art therapy has been successfully pursued for the benefit of those involved: terminal illness, cancer, child abuse, suicide (especially among teenagers), high-risk pregnancy, and coping with loss.

People are also beginning to explore the benefits of full-spectrum lighting in managing conditions caused by light deprivation in northern climes.

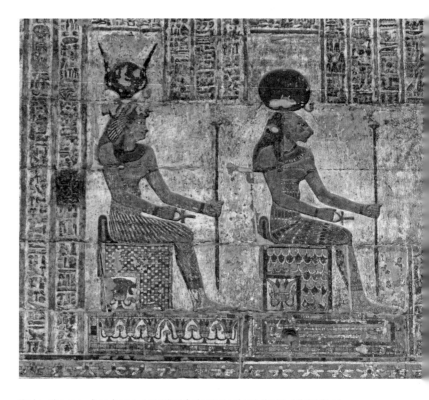

Color therapy has been practiced since ancient times. Historians believe that the Egyptians chose particular colors to decorate their temples, tombs, and sanctuaries for the effects that they produce psychologically, spiritually, and perhaps physically.

Color Therapy

Color therapists associate the spectrum of colors with an energy field or "aura" surrounding the body. When you feel unwell, one or more of your energy fields may be off-balance. Therapists use the color appropriate to the affected region to help restore balance and well-being. The color may be introduced in a number of ways, including wearing clothing of the appropriate color, by vizualization techniques during meditation, or by eating foods of a particular color.

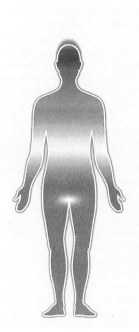

Violet

Violet relates to the crown and top of the head, energizing the pituitary gland and stimulating the upper brain and nervous system. Spiritually calming and anti-inflammatory, its inspirational qualities promote meditation and visualization, relieve sinus congestion and headaches, and may help in conditions such as multiple sclerosis. Violet should be avoided as a therapy for the mentally ill and when experiencing alcohol and drug problems.

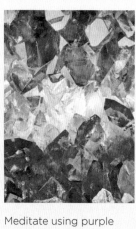

Meditate using purple flowers and gemstones as your focus, use lavender oils, and eat red cabbage, grapes, and figs.

Indigo

Indigo stimulates the imagination and intuition, calms the nerves, aids insomnia, and eases migraine. It should not be used in cases of mental illness, when suffering from eating disorders, or when prescribed sedatives.

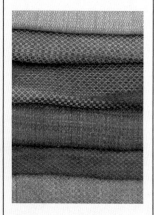

Wear more indigo and dark blue clothes, focus your meditation on gemstones of this color, and eat eggplants, beets, and plums.

Blue

Blue corresponds to the thyroid gland, throat, and base of the skull. As an anti-inflammatory color, blue can calm nerves and promote peace, relieve sunburn or wounds, and ease throat, voice, and neck problems. An excess of blue should be avoided if you are trying to keep warm or when suffering from thyroid deficiency.

Focus on the blue sky and sea during meditation, use lavender oils, and eat blueberries, plums, and grapes.

Green

Green corresponds to the thymus gland, heart, lungs, and immune system. It brings harmony and tranquility, relieves breathing problems, and calms anxiety. It should be avoided when suffering from autoimmunity problems when logical analysis is required.

Yellow

Yellow corresponds to the areas of the adrenal glands, solar plexus, and digestive and circulatory systems. Increasing the amount of yellow in your surroundings will ease mental fatigue, aid digestion, relax muscles, and combat nervousness. Avoid yellow when suffering from hyperactivity, stomachache, or if prone to aggressive behavior.

Orange

Orange is an energy-giving color that covers the middle section of the body, including the kidneys, abdomen, and lower back. Increased vitality, relief from urinary and menstrual problems, and improved appetite may be achieved by using orange. Avoid orange if you are of an irritable disposition, suffer from intestinal problems, or would like to relax.

Red

Red corresponds to the lower body, from the base of the spine and hips down to the feet, and includes the reproductive organs. Use it to increase physical stamina, relieve lower back pain, and improve circulation. Avoid red if you have high blood pressure, heart problems, or when relaxation is your aim.

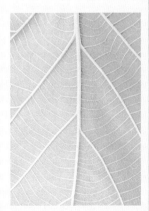

Fill your home with green plants, spend more time in the garden, eat avocados, spinach, and salad leaves, and use pine and bergamot oils.

Meditate using yellow as your focus, use citronella and lemon oils, and eat bananas, corn, eggs, and yellow spices such as turmeric.

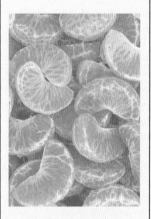

Wear orange clothing, eat tangerines, carrots, and ginseng, and visualize orange.

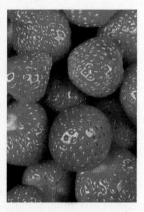

Wear red garments, eat tomatoes, strawberries, and cherries, and use oils such as myrrh and patchouli.

BIOFEEDBACK

Biofeedback is a technique by which we can detect biological information from our own bodies. It can demonstrate to us that changes in internal processes occurring from moment to moment are the result of mental and emotional changes we can learn to control. This is called self-regulation. Once we have learned self-regulation and voluntary control of any internal state, that ability is ours for life.

A biofeedback meter enables people to monitor changes that affect their blood pressure and see the effect of modifying techniques.

Biological feedback has been known for over a century, but it was not until the 1960s that pioneering efforts by Dr. Elmer Green led other researchers to develop the potential of this remarkable technology and apply it to human ailments. It has also been a valuable tool in the development of psychoneuro-immunology, which studies the precise mechanisms by which we turn thoughts and feelings into chemical and neurological sequences in the body.

Using safe and simple devices, biofeedback gives the subject instant information about any number of body processes. The subject uses that information to adjust a function that is under his or her control, thereby altering the body process that is being observed.

Here is one example. A person subject to high blood pressure has a tiny cuff attached to a finger. The cuff measures peripheral blood flow (a factor that is abnormal in high blood pressure). The little cuff is attached to a flow meter that the subject can watch constantly. He or she is taught to breathe properly and to relax all the muscle groups in the body. These methods are known to make peripheral blood flow more normal. By watching the flow meter, the effect of the method can be monitored and the information loop is now complete.

All the person needs to do now is use the method at home at prescribed intervals to make the needle move in the right direction so that the blood pressure tends toward normal. He or she has made an objective link between relaxation and blood pressure that is undeniable. Not only does the method help to relieve high blood pressure, which can be

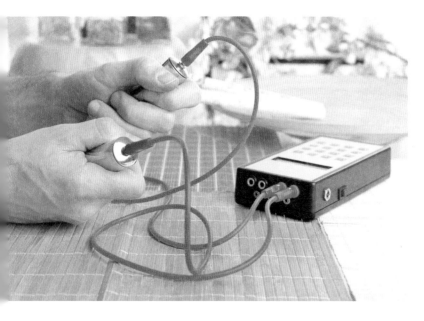

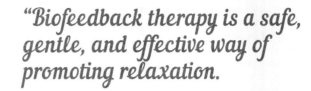

"Biofeedback therapy is a safe, gentle, and effective way of promoting relaxation.

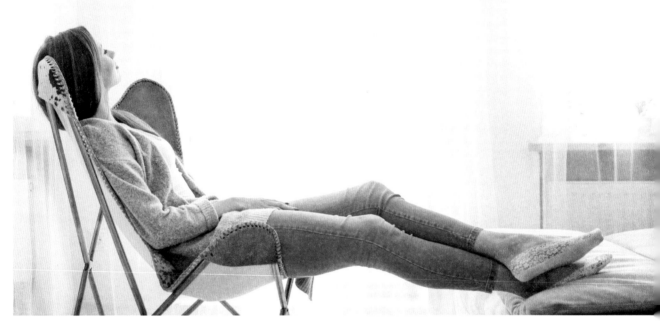

dangerous, but it also shows the subject a lot about how the body works and how we can consciously regulate many of its internal functions.

There are many possible biofeedback applications.

Feedback of skin conductance and breathing: In addition to peripheral blood flow, this allows us to gain awareness, then modulation, of various autonomic processes, including those connected with the heart and circulation, breathing, and digestive and hormonal responses. In this way, we can gain some control of headaches, blood pressure, heart rate and rhythm, ulcers, irritable bowel, pain, anger, anxiety, and panic.

Neuromuscular feedback: This enables many people to reduce muscle spasm and then to regain the use of the weakened muscles.

Brain wave neurofeedback: This helps normalize brain functions, enhances creativity, greatly improves attention and concentration, and alleviates cravings and addictions.

When one considers that all of these disorders are conventionally treated by expensive and potentially toxic drugs and surgery, this approach has much to commend it, especially in a climate in which toxicity and expense are becoming bigger medical issues every day.

While there is still resistance to the idea of biofeedback, it is more appealing to the scientific mind than many complementary therapies. This is probably because it has a dial on a conventional apparatus that can measure something changing, and that change can itself be measured and monitored.

A simple biofeedback device can help train the mind to control the body. It allows you to see just how effective different relaxation techniques are by monitoring changes in blood pressure.

THERAPIES RELATING TO THE WORLD AROUND US

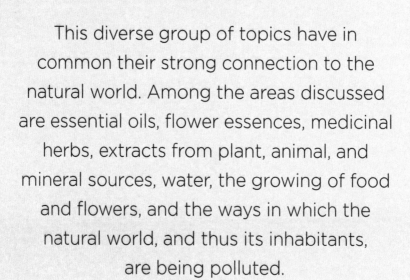

This diverse group of topics have in common their strong connection to the natural world. Among the areas discussed are essential oils, flower essences, medicinal herbs, extracts from plant, animal, and mineral sources, water, the growing of food and flowers, and the ways in which the natural world, and thus its inhabitants, are being polluted.

HYDROTHERAPY

Since early times, water has been recognized as having therapeutic, even miraculous, properties. From the Roman and Turkish baths, through Bavaria, Britain, and Lourdes, to modern saunas and physiotherapy departments, hydrotherapy has consistently proved its value.

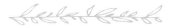

There are many ways in which water can be used therapeutically.

Externally: Water can be used in the form of baths, douches, and packs.

Baths: These wash away sweat, combat inflammation by stimulating blood circulation, and exert tonic and soothing effects on the emotional system. Cold baths have an invigorating effect as well. Hot baths can be the medium for adding various substances to water, such as salts, minerals, and herbs. Baths of intermediate temperature (90-95°F/32-35°C) can last much longer than hot or cold baths and are effective in reducing tension. Whirlpool and aerated bathtubs have specific uses. Sitz baths, in which one sits in a basin or bathtub of appropriate size and shape, are especially useful for abdominal, pelvic, and genitourinary problems, by bringing blood selectively to that part of the body.

A douche: This is a strong stream of water directed locally or generally on the body. We are most familiar with the ordinary shower. The effects of douches are similar to those of baths, with the advantage of the mechanical effects of jets or sprays.

Packs and compresses: These can be used hot or cold, depending on the effect desired. Ice packs have a quick and direct effect that is useful in the aftermath of injury, when they can minimize swelling and bleeding into the tissues.

Internally: Water can be used in the form of enemas and colonic irrigations, for removing waste products and toxins. It can also be inhaled as vapor and steam, which helps to cleanse the respiratory tract.

Hydrotherapy treatment in whirlpool bathtubs that massage and stimulate the body with pressurized jets can be used to treat ailments and promote relaxation.

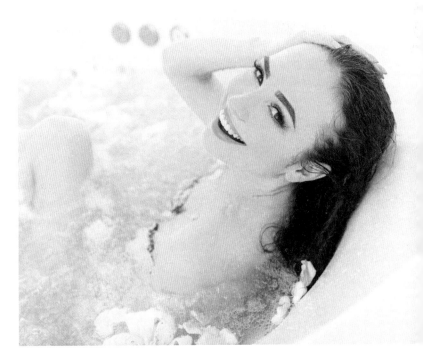

AROMATHERAPY

The therapeutic use of essential oils can be traced back thousands of years to the early Egyptian empire. Aromatic oils were known in biblical times. We know from numerous writings that they were valued in many ancient cultures in the Middle and Far East, including Greece, Arabia, China, and India.

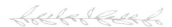

Aromatherapy oils are usually diluted in a carrier oil before application to the skin.

The distillation of essential oils is thought to have been discovered in the 10th century by an Arab physician known to us as Avicenna. For the past few centuries, the world's essential oil industry has been centered in Grasse, in southern France, and much modern research has been done by French chemists. One of these, René-Maurice Gattefosse, did important healing work with wounded soldiers in World War I and he later coined the term aromatherapy.

Since that time, it has been established without doubt that essential oils are absorbed through the skin into the circulatory system and distributed to the body cells, a process that takes between 30 minutes and 12 hours. By massage and in baths are the preferred methods of application to the skin. Inhalation is even more direct. It carries the oil to the olfactory nerves, which transmit the effects directly to the brain, where intuition, emotion, and creativity can be affected extremely quickly. Less often, essential oils are taken orally on a sugar cube.

The extraction of oils is complex and expensive to perform, being both time- and labor-intensive and requiring expensive equipment. Huge amounts of plant stock are required to distill minute quantities of oil—for example, it takes 250lb (350kg) of rose petals to produce 1oz (30g) of essential oil. For these reasons, it is not worth trying to extract essential oils at home.

Aromatherapy, as it is usually practiced, is a blending of massage, herbal therapy, hydrotherapy, reflexology, and even Bach flower essence theory with the essential oils used. There are at least 40 oils in common use. Readily available from stores and supply houses, they have differing properties and combinations of properties: antiseptic, warming, cooling, astringent, stimulating, soothing, relaxing, sedative, decongestant, antispasmodic, and so on.

It is best to take instruction from someone experienced in the use of essential oils if you wish to become proficient and knowledgeable about the subject. Certain cautions need to be observed, such as oils that should be avoided when treating some people or conditions, and these need to be learned.

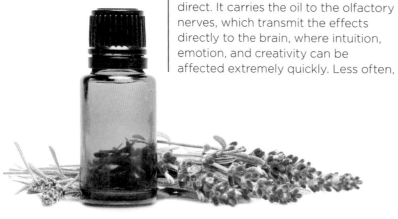

Diluting Essential Oils

If using aromatherapy oils for massage, they should be diluted in a carrier oil first. Cold-pressed vegetable oils make the best base. Peach, apricot, sweet almond, grapeseed, sunflower, and safflower oils are all very good. If using olive or wheatgerm oil, dilute the oil with another, lighter variety as the smell of these oils on their own can be overpowering. Coconut oil is probably the lightest oil of all and is therefore particularly appropriate for milder, floral-based essential oils.

Another consideration is that both oils and essences will oxidize with time. If you decide to mix a quantity of oil for future use, store it in a dark, airtight glass bottle and keep the bottle in a cool, dry place out of the reach of sunlight. The refrigerator is a good storage place. Adding a little wheatgerm oil to the mixture will slow down the process of oxidation but will not prevent it, so do not mix too large a quantity—you will only have to throw it away.

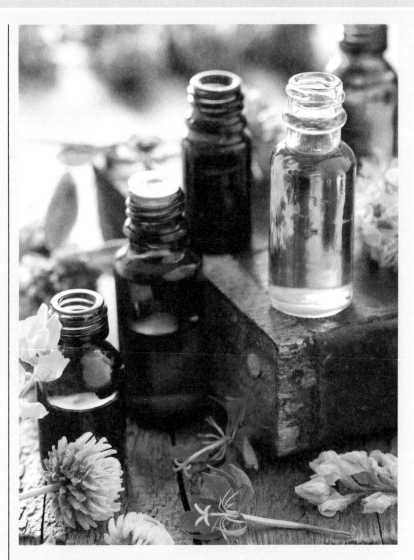

Mixing the oils

- If you want to use essential oils in a bath, simply put around five drops directly into the water.

- If using the oil directly on the body, add around 20 drops of essential oil to 2oz (50ml) of carrier oil.

- If using the oil directly on the face, put 10 drops of essential oil in 2oz (50ml) of carrier oil.

- For children, reduce the quantity of essential oil to 5–10 drops.

- If burning essential oils, put around five drops in the oil holder and fill up with water.

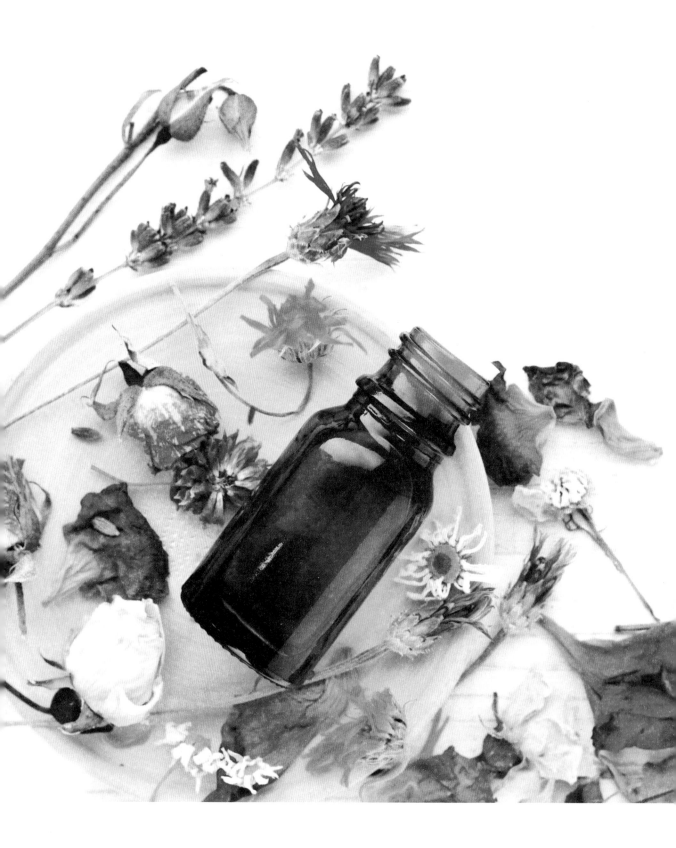

Aromatherapy Oils

■ **Basil**
ear problems

■ **Benzoin**
cough, sore throat

■ **Bergamot**
cold sores, depression, menopausal problems, skin symptoms

■ **Black pepper**
headache, toothache, circulatory problems

■ **Cajuput**
ear inflammation

■ **Cedarwood**
dry cough

■ **Chamomile**
ear problems, strengthening gums, dry cough, eczema, insomnia, menstural problems, soft tissue symptoms

■ **Cinnamon**
cold symptoms

■ **Clary sage**
anxiety, insomnia

■ **Clove**
toothache, nausea, and vomiting

■ **Cypress**
acne, varicose veins, intestinal and urinary problems

■ **Eucalyptus**
headache, cold symptoms, breathlessness, cold sores, cough, hay fever

■ **Fennel**
strengthening gums, intestinal problems

■ **Frankincense**
breathlessness

■ **Geranium**
diarrhea, eczema, ringworm, acne, depression, anxiety and panic

■ **Ginger**
sore throat, dry cough, morning sickness

■ **Grapefruit**
colds and flu

■ **Honey water**
nausea

■ **Hyssop**
ear problems

■ **Jasmine**
depression, menopausal problems

■ **Juniper**
toothache, diarrhea, acne, circulatory problems

■ **Lavender**
headache, ear problems, breathlessness, heartburn, eczema, athlete's foot, ringworm, bites and stings, insomnia, anxiety and panic, depression, circulatory problems, cold sores, earache

■ **Lemon**
acne, athlete's foot, depression, cystitis, flu symptoms, nosebleed, sore throat

■ **Marjoram**
headache, arthritis, menstrual problems, circulatory problems

■ **Melissa**
headache, anxiety and panic, menstrual problems

■ **Myrrh**
strengthening gums, athlete's foot

■ **Neroli**
insomnia, anxiety and panic, depression, skin symptoms, impotence

■ **Orange**
depression

■ **Patchouli**
anxiety and panic

■ **Peppermint**
headache, toothache, cold and flu symptoms, nausea and vomiting, diarrhea, fainting

■ **Pettigrain**
fainting

■ **Pine**
hay fever, sinus headache, incontinence

■ **Rose**
headache, ear problems, insomnia, anxiety and panic, depression, eczema, sunburn, menstrual problems

■ **Rosemary**
headache, head lice, arthritis, intestinal problems, circulatory problems

■ **Sage**
strengthening gums, toothache, breathlessness

■ **Sandalwood**
sore throat, anxiety and panic, cystitis, impotence

■ **Savory**
ear problems

■ **Sweet marjoram**
insomnia

■ **Tea tree**
sore throat, cold symptoms, athlete's foot, ringworm, cold sores, headlice, bites and stings, skin symptoms

■ **Thyme**
cough, sore throat, sinus headache

■ **Ylang-ylang**
anxiety and panic, depression

■ **Wheatgerm**
sunburn

BACH FLOWER REMEDIES

The simple and natural method of healing that bears his name was discovered by Edward Bach, a renowned physician and bacteriologist, who practiced in London for over 20 years. In 1919 he was profoundly impressed by the concepts and work of Samuel Christian Hahnemann, the founder of homeopathy (see page 244). In 1930 he left his lucrative medical practice behind and went to Wales to immerse himself in the world of plants.

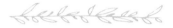

Chicory is one of the 38 plants included in Edward Bach's method of healing.

He became convinced, through a combination of intuition and experimentation, that while many plants had medicinal properties to soothe and relieve suffering, a certain few plants contained true healing power—that is, the capacity to restore health to mind and body. He set out to discover exactly which plants possessed this power. He knew they had to be common plants, not toxic or harmful in any way, and developed what he felt was the ideal method of extracting the essence of the plant, by placing the perfectly formed petals of the flower on the surface of fresh water in the sun. After many months of sensing and experimenting, he narrowed the field to 38 plants that he grouped as follows, according to the predominant moods and states of mind in which he found their effect to be beneficial.

Fear: Rock rose, mimulus, aspen, red chestnut, and cherry plum

Loneliness: Water violet, impatiens, and heather

Oversensitivity to influences and ideas: Agrimony, centaury, walnut, and holly

Despondency or despair: Larch, pine, elm, sweet chestnut, star of Bethlehem, willow, oak, and crab apple

Uncertainty: Cerato, scleranthus, gentian, gorse, hornbeam, and wild oat

Insufficient interest in present circumstances: Clematis, honeysuckle, wild rose, olive, white chestnut, mustard, and chestnut bud

Over-concern for welfare of others: Chicory, vervain, vine, beech, and rock water

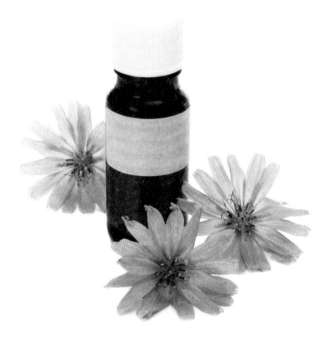

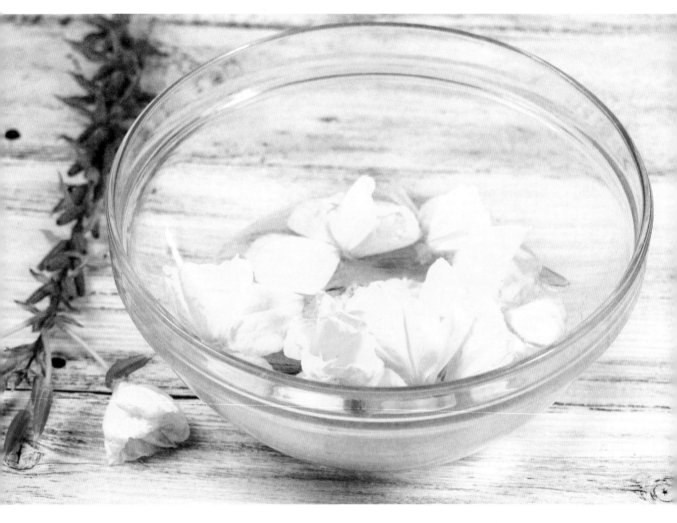

In order to prescribe, you need the booklet *The Twelve Healers* to ascertain which remedy is appropriate to individual states of mind, as there are many variations within each grouping. The Bach flower remedies are available individually and in the complete set. Rescue Remedy, a selection of five remedies that is used to deal with everyday emergencies, is probably the most well known. They are absolutely benign in their action and can never produce an unpleasant reaction.

It was Bach's intention that they could be safely prescribed and used by anyone. The essences are usually preserved using brandy, but for those who are sensitive to alcohol, the brandy can be omitted—the essence will just not remain preserved for as long. To become proficient in prescribing for yourself or others, you need to become adept at observing mental attitudes and moods. A good understanding can be obtained from reading about the subject. The actual dispensing is quite easy—you just follow simple directions.

Bach flower remedies are derived from petals placed on spring water and exposed to the sun.

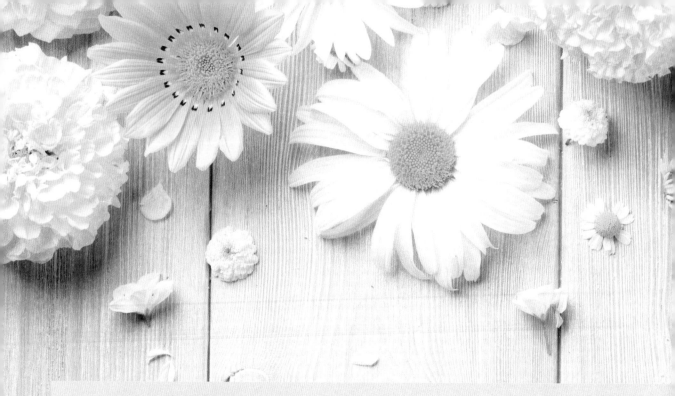

Bach Flower Remedies

■ Agrimony
encourages those who hide worries behind a cheerful face to express anxieties

■ Aspen
allays feelings of fear due to unknown cause

■ Beech
encourages tolerance in those who are overcritical

■ Centaury
helps those who are unassertive to discover and achieve what they want

■ Cerato
helps those who doubt their own judgment to trust in themselves

■ Cherry plum
reassures those who feel near to breakdown

■ Chestnut bud
helps those who repeatedly make the same mistakes to learn from them instead

■ Chicory
enables those who are overpossessive to let go

■ Clematis
aids concentration and focuses the mind

■ Crabapple
known as "the cleanser", this helps those with negative feelings of self-disgust to put everything into perspective

■ Elm
restores confidence to those who feel overwhelmed

■ Gentian
gives renewed faith in life to those who are despondent

■ Gorse
restores hope in those who feel despair

■ Heather
develops compassion in those who are self-obsessed

■ Holly
dampens negative emotions of jealousy and envy

■ Honeysuckle
helps those who are nostalgic for the past to let go and live in the present

■ Hornbeam
known as "Monday morning" remedy, this restores energy

■ Impatiens
encourages patience and tolerance

■ Larch
enhances self-confidence and lessens fear of failure

■ Mimulus
helps those who are afraid of specific things to deal with those fears and phobias

■ Mustard
instils optimism in those who feel despair

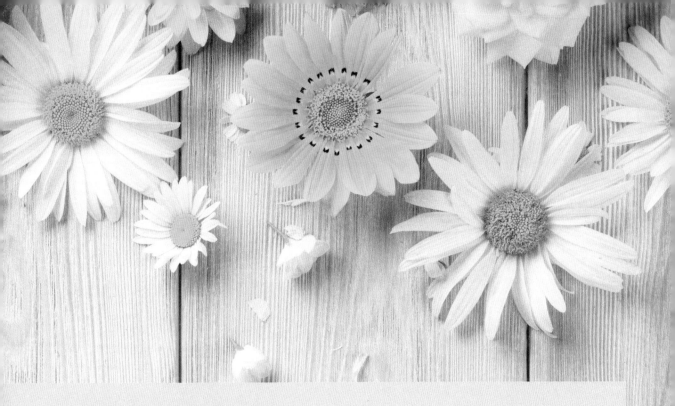

- **Oak**
rebuilds strength and endurance in those who normally overachieve but can no longer cope

- **Olive**
regenerates peace and balance after hardship

- **Pine**
helps those with a guilt complex to forgive themselves

- **Red chestnut**
helps those who are over-solicitous of others to put fears into perspective

- **Rock rose**
gives courage to those who are afraid and alarmed

- **Rock water**
helps those who are too rigid to be more lenient toward themselves

- **Schleranthus**
improves indecision and uncertainty

- **Star of Bethlehem**
reassures after shock

- **Sweet chestnut**
gives hope to those in deep despair

- **Vervain**
restores balance to those with fanatical tendencies

- **Vine**
encourages those who are authoritarian to be more understanding of others

- **Walnut**
protects those who are undergoing periods of change

- **Water violet**
helps those who are withdrawn and reserved to open up to others

- **White chestnut**
restores peace of mind and dispels unwanted thoughts

- **Wild oat**
encourages decisiveness and clears confusion

- **Wild rose**
gives motivation and dispels feelings of apathy

- **Willow**
encourages positive frame of mind in those who feel bitter

- **Rescue remedy**
combination of cherry plum, clematis, impatiens, rock rose, and star of Bethlehem; comforts and calms in times of emergency and stress

HERBAL THERAPY

Herbal therapy has been practiced for thousands of years and still takes place in every corner of the globe. Virtually every one of the last 40 centuries has had noted practitioners of the art. In scores of cultures today, herbalism is a prominent feature of society.

You can make tea bags by wrapping your herbs in gauze or cheesecloth to avoid having to strain an infusion.

Many "modern" drugs are derived from plant sources. Yet in the mainstream of Western technological society, herbalism has been shunted into the background. Today there seems to be a shift in this tide, as drug researchers are venturing into remote areas of the world in search of native remedies they might use and market.

Meanwhile, many thousands of people are benefiting from the accumulated knowledge of the centuries, both for their health and their culinary enrichment. In this book we focus on the healthy aspects of herbs, for which the term "herbal therapy" is not an exaggeration. (Some authors use the term "botanical medicine.") Herbs or their products are available for virtually every symptom discussed in this book. Space permits touching only on certain aspects of their diversity and richness.

Herbs are simply plants possessing special qualities beneficial to humans and animals. You can grow many of them yourself, either for consumption or for medicinal use, in a yard or even in pots on the windowsill. Those you cannot grow can be purchased either locally or online. It is a good rule never to use a plant from your garden or from the wild that you have not positively identified.

If you grow or gather plants, you will want to dry some for later use. Pick them in the morning and either spread them out in a thin layer on a clean surface or hang them in an airy place in bunches, taking care to disturb them as little as possible. For storing, use airtight jars made of dark glass or airtight cans. Keep them in a cool, dry place for no longer than a year. This is a handy interval for growing and gathering a fresh supply. Many herbs can also be frozen.

Herbal products are prepared in several ways. The only preparations that can be kept for any length of time are ointments and those made with alcohol. The following products are those most commonly used in herbal therapy.

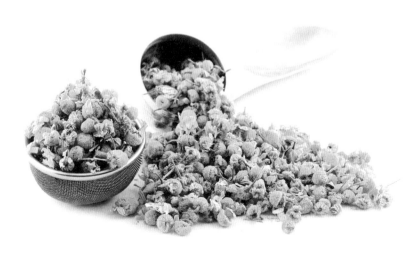

Infusions: The plant is combined with boiling water and steeped for about 10 minutes, strained into a glass or cup, and sweetened with a little honey to make a beverage like tea.

Decoctions: These are similar to infusions but use bark roots and similar ingredients.

Juicing: Fresh plants and plant parts are chopped up and pressed to squeeze out the juice to extract the water-soluble parts. This is an excellent way of getting vitamins and minerals from the plant.

Powder: Dried plant parts are ground with a mortar and pestle until powdered, and then taken with liquids, sprinkled on food, put into capsules, and so on.

Syrup: Herbal ingredients are added to honey or brown sugar in water, boiled, and then strained. This method is good for administration to children.

Tincture: Powdered herb is added to a 50 percent alcohol solution and allowed to stand for two weeks, shaken daily, then strained and bottled.

Ointment: Powdered herb is added to hot petroleum jelly.

Poultice: Crushed plant parts are mixed with hot moist flour or cornmeal, or a mixture of bread and milk, to make a warm paste. This is then applied to the skin. It is covered with a cloth and kept moist with warm water at intervals. It is also known as a plaster.

Cold compress: A cloth is soaked in a cooled infusion and applied to an affected part.

Herb baths: See Hydrotherapy on page 231.

Herbs have been an important source of fragrance and healing for centuries.

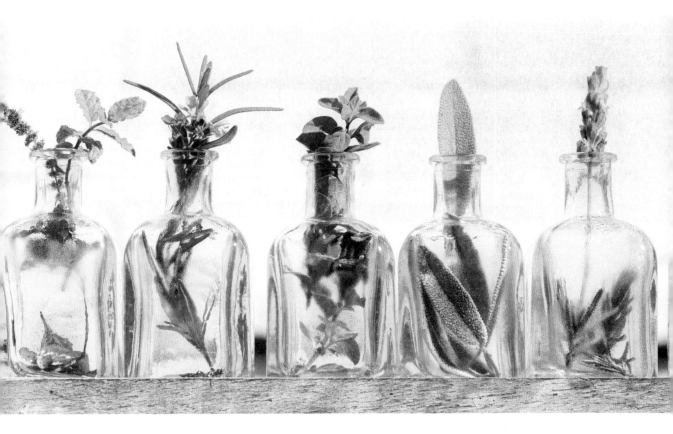

Herbal Remedies

- **Aloe vera**
cough

- **Arnica**
pain, immune disorders

- **Astragalus**
fatigue, immune disorders

- **Basil**
depression

- **Belladonna**
abdominal pain

- **Butcher's broom**
anal/genital symptoms

- **Calendula**
eye problems, abdominal and intestinal problems

- **Caraway**
halitosis

- **Cardamom**
indigestion

- **Catnip**
headache

- **Cayenne pepper**
joint pain

- **Chamomile**
eye problems, abdominal problems, insomnia

- **Chickweed**
eye problems, skin disorders

- **Cinnamon**
abdominal pain

- **Clove**
toothache

- **Coltsfoot**
cough, diarrhea

- **Comfrey**
skin disorders

- **Cranesbill**
anal/genital symptoms

- **Cucumber**
eye problems

- **Dandelion**
eye problems, indigestion, menstrual disorders

- **Dill**
halitosis, indigestion

- **Echinacea**
headache, ear and throat problems, infections, immune disorders

- **Elderflower**
eye problems, cold symptoms, skin disorders

- **Ephedra**
breathlessness

- **European centaury**
appetite stimulation

- **Fennel**
sinus, bronchitis, abdominal pain, indigestion

- **Fenugreek**
diabetic symptoms

- **Feverfew**
joint pain, migraine

- **Garlic**
headache, diarrhea, infections, high cholesterol

- **Ginger**
chronic pain, indigestion

- **Ginseng**
fatigue

- **Goldenseal**
headache, indigestion, loss of appetite

- **Gum guggula**
high cholesterol

- **Hawthorn**
dizziness, hypertension

- **St. John's wort**
back pain, chronic pain, depression, anorexia

- **Hyssop**
coughs

- **Juniper berries**
appetite stimulation

- **Lavender**
headache, dizziness, cramps

- **Lemon balm**
abdominal pain, insomnia

- **Licorice**
bronchitis, addictions

- **Lime blossom**
insomnia, depression

- **Marigold**
eye problems, sore throat, menstrual disorders

- **Meadowsweet**
fever, diarrhea, chronic pain

- **Motherwort**
menstrual disorders

- **Nettle**
menstrual disorders, appetite stimulation

- **Parsley**
menstrual disorders

- **Passionflower**
insomnia

- **Peppermint**
dizziness, indigestion, cold symptoms, nausea, diarrhea, abdominal pain, indigestion

- **Red eyebright**
eye problems

- **Red sage**
sore throat

- **Rosemary**
indigestion, jaundice

- **Rue**
headache, dizziness

- **Sage**
dizziness

- **Sandalwood**
fever, urinary symptoms

- **Slippery elm**
ear and throat problems, joint pain, indigestion

- **Tansy**
ear and throat problems

- **Thyme**
coughs, breathlessness

- **Valerian**
back pain

- **Willow**
ear and throat problems

- **Yarrow**
headache, colds

Making an infusion

An infusion is a kind of tea made by steeping herbs in hot water. It is most suitable for leaves and flowers. Put two teaspoonfuls per person of the herb or herbal mixture in a warmed glass or china teapot and add two cupfuls of boiling water. Leave to infuse for about 10 minutes, stirring occasionally. Strain the infusion into a cup and sweeten with a little honey if you wish. Infusions can be drunk hot, cold, or iced.

Making a poultice

A poultice, or plaster, can be used to apply herbs externally to an affected area. Mix the crushed herbs into a warm paste of flour or cornmeal and water, or bread and milk, apply to the skin and cover with a cloth. Keep moist by the addition of warm water at intervals. The herbs can also be mixed with a little warm water and placed between layers of gauze or cheesecloth before application to the skin.

Making a decoction

A decoction is used for the hard parts of the plant, such as roots, bark, and seeds, which must be boiled or simmered to release their essences. Add 1oz (30g) of the herbal mixture to each 16oz (500ml) of water in a pan. Do not use an aluminum pan, which will leach toxic traces into the mixture. Bring to a boil and simmer for about 10 minutes. Cool and strain, squeezing the herbs in order to extract all the juices.

Making a tincture

A tincture is a way of preserving herbs for up to about two years. This is usually done in alcohol, which is also a good solvent for most of the active substances in the herb. Tinctures from a herbal supplier tend to be stronger and last longer, but they can be homemade by adding powdered herb to a 50 percent alcohol solution. Leave to steep for two weeks, shaking daily, strain, and bottle. Add a tablespoonful to water or tea.

HOMEOPATHY

Homeopathy is the system of medicine discovered and developed by Samuel Christian Hahnemann in the late 18th and early 19th centuries. From reading and observation he discovered the principle that "like is healed by like," meaning that the symptoms produced in the body by a substance, such as quinine, are similar to the symptoms that the substance is used to alleviate.

Homeopathic remedies for many symptoms are readily available for self-treatment.

Another of Hahnemann's discoveries was that the effect of a remedy is made more potent by repeated dilutions. A third discovery was that by shaking or agitating a solution in a certain way (a process called succussion), the potency of the preparation is further enhanced.

A homeopathic physician is trained as extensively as a conventional, or allopathic, physician. In fact a high proportion of those who practice homeopathy are also fully trained in conventional medicine. The homeopath must understand all aspects of disease, pharmacology, and pharmacotherapy, and must be capable of seeing the barriers between the patient and good health. Fortunately, homeopathic preparations are available to individuals for the treatment of virtually all symptoms. They are most accessible in health food stores. These products are labeled according to the symptoms for which they are to be taken and they are generally safe to use.

The manufacture of homeopathic products is very complicated. They are made from plant, animal, and other biological sources, and from mineral sources. After extraction and filtration, tinctures are made to which minerals are added. It is after that stage that the serial dilutions take place, followed by succussion. Preparations include tablets, granules, ointments, liquids, and suppositories.

Many people have become acquainted with, and gained confidence in, homeopathic theory and practice, though far fewer people practice homeopathy than conventional medicine. As a consequence, a large percentage of those who use homeopathy do so without ever seeing a homeopathic practitioner, but simply purchase preparations, or "remedies," and use them at home. This works well for many symptoms, such as headache, abdominal cramps, cough, or insomnia, but for more deep-rooted and persistent symptoms, many find themselves seeking out a homeopathic physician to go through the more complicated process of sorting out the symptoms and prescribing remedies.

NATUROPATHY

Naturopathic medicine has roots that go far back in world history, and it embodies practices from many differing cultural origins. For nearly a century, it has been a distinct entity in American medicine; it now has its own medical colleges, where a rigorous program is pursued that rivals that of the allopathic model. Each year, more states are added to the list of places in which naturopathic practice is licensed.

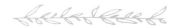

The basic principles of naturopathy are based on the concept that the body is a self-healing organism. Naturopathic physicians enhance the body's own healing responses through noninvasive measures and health promotion. They treat both acute and chronic diseases using nutrition, herbal or botanical medicine, homeopathy, traditional Chinese medicine, physical medicine, exercise therapy, counseling, and hydrotherapy.

Naturopathic treatment might include a short, juice-only fast to cleanse the body and promote self-healing.

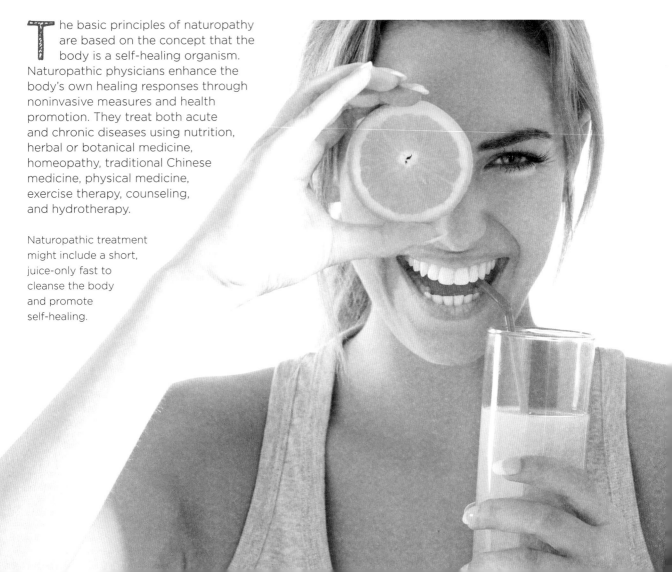

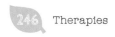

GARDENING AND GROWING

The cycle of planting, tending, and harvesting is an important way for us to connect with the earth and the realm of beings on whom we depend for much of our nourishment. The basis for discussing it as a therapy is that it is a self-healing activity that one can perform on one's own plot of ground. This connection seems entirely appropriate.

The joy of seeing buds unfurl in spring is part of the therapy of gardening.

One of the things that has been alarming about the process of industrialization and urbanization that has taken place in the last few centuries is that there are now many millions of people who have little knowledge or understanding of the processes that put food on our table or the way of life which supports that.

Another aspect of this shift in the life of our culture is the demise of the family in favor of the huge agri-businesses that now produce most of our food. Some of the negative aspects of this, such as toxicity and soil depletion, are touched upon in Combating Environmental Pollution on page 248.

The positive side of this is that many people are discovering health and satisfaction in varying degrees of gardening and growing activities. The only distinction drawn here between gardening and growing is the extent of the endeavor (small kitchen garden vs. an acre of corn). Even in suburban areas, there is a resurgence of individual and community gardens. The proliferation of farmers' markets and the advent of even higher standards for the labeling of food as "organic" are particularly good signs. Many people are producing more food than they need and selling the excess at or to the local farmers' market. The upgrading of produce in the chain stores, a response to local competition, is an excellent ripple effect of this which means that an ever wider circle of people has access to nutritious food.

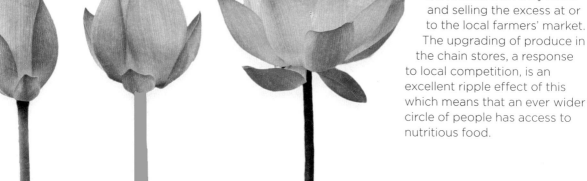

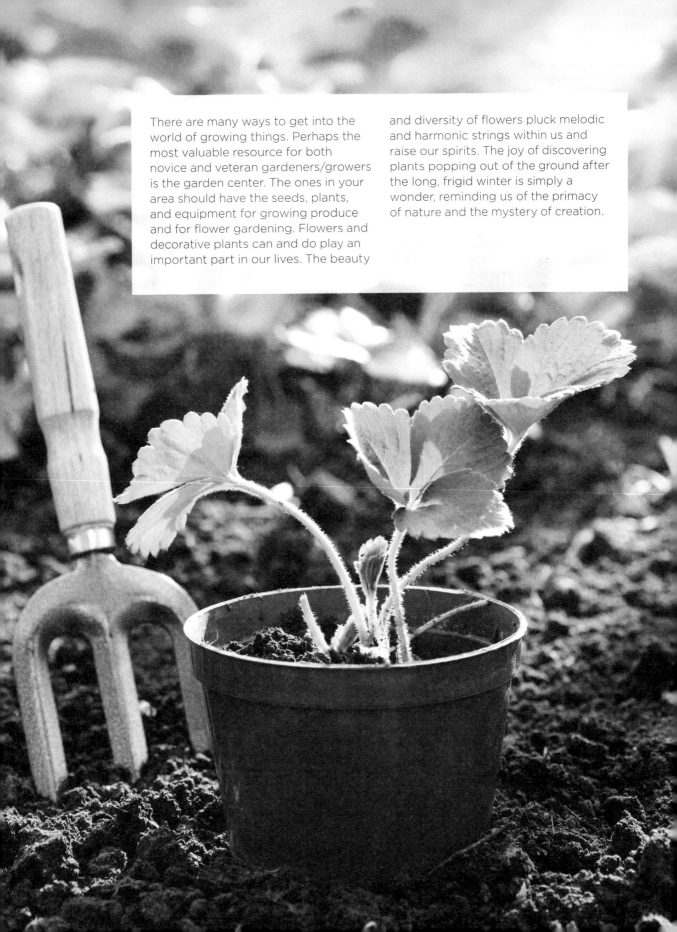

There are many ways to get into the world of growing things. Perhaps the most valuable resource for both novice and veteran gardeners/growers is the garden center. The ones in your area should have the seeds, plants, and equipment for growing produce and for flower gardening. Flowers and decorative plants can and do play an important part in our lives. The beauty and diversity of flowers pluck melodic and harmonic strings within us and raise our spirits. The joy of discovering plants popping out of the ground after the long, frigid winter is simply a wonder, reminding us of the primacy of nature and the mystery of creation.

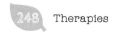

COMBATING ENVIRONMENTAL POLLUTION

It has become increasingly clear in the past few decades that certain elements in our physical environment constitute a real threat to our health. We should all become conversant with the issues involved, to help us formulate effective strategies and to take action aimed at making the planet once again a safe and healthy place to live.

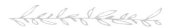

This is clearly as important to our future as a society as other steps we take that primarily affect our personal inner environment.

Air pollution: We are constantly under threat from those who pollute the air and from those who would strip away the hard-won gains that have been made in the battle against pollution. Among the conditions that are directly attributable to air pollution are emphysema, sinus trouble, allergies, infections, skin conditions, and some cancers. Many other conditions are also caused by air pollution, either directly or indirectly.

Water pollution and scarcity: Regional scarcity of water is partially due to migration of people to warm, sunny climes, where water is already in short supply. This is complicated by the inappropriate uses to which water is put in these areas, such as maintaining lawns in arid zones when using indigenous plants would make a lot more sense. Scarcity aggravates the already major problem of water pollution by chemicals such as chlorine. Chemical pollution of water is known to contribute to cancer, allergies, and diseases of the nervous system and respiratory tract.

Food chain degradation: The use of pesticides, antibiotics, and chemical fertilizers, which is particularly prevalent in the agri-business of today, is a large demonstrable factor in the breakdown of health in the early 21st century, a time in which there is longer life but greater ill-health. Food allergies, for example, once virtually unknown, have been on the increase for a generation, as has infection with yeasts and fungi. These conditions, which affect millions, are directly related to modern agricultural practices. These practices result in marked demineralization of the soil, and food that is deficient in the nutrients we need to remain healthy and whole. We are thus increasingly dependent on supplements to provide our basic nutritional needs.

"The quality of the air we breathe in our personal environment can be improved by a humidifier or ionizer."

Population explosion: This is one of the most sensitive issues on the political landscape, as it touches people's lives in so many personal ways. It intersects the issues of abortion, adoption, free choice, and sexual freedom in the arenas of economics, politics, and individual rights. Population increase has become so great that it amounts to a global crisis—the time that it takes to double the world's population has dropped from centuries to just a few years. Until about 1980, it could be stated that feeding the world's people was only a matter of distribution. However, we can no longer make that claim—now there is not enough food being produced to feed the world's people and their numbers are increasing all the time.

Electrical and radiation pollution: As recently as a century ago, there were virtually no man-made electromagnetic or radiation emanations present in the atmosphere. Now our environment is charged with a phenomenal variety of emanations: radio, telephone, short-wave, television, computers, X-ray screening (diagnosis and therapy), scanning technology, and satellite projects—the list goes on and on. There is a growing body of evidence linking these developments to human illness.

This is not surprising when one considers the number of electrical systems operating within us that can be tampered with by outside emanations: the heart, the brain, all the nerves, all the muscles, all the body fluids carrying charged particles to and from the cells. That pretty well covers the whole body!

Having stated the problems, we must resolve to look at the subject of environmental pollution in a positive light—what can we do, individually and collectively, to make a positive impact on these various areas? The following suggestions are among those that come to mind.

- Learn more about these areas, so that we can pass information on to others with confidence.
- Spread the word to as many people as possible. When enough people have the information that we have, a threshold will be crossed and something good will happen. It has been stated that when as few as one percent of people have had their awareness raised, then their combined positivity is enough to influence the whole of society.
- Learn how to be a political activist for the environment. Legislators really do respond to what their constituents say and think, even if they only see it as a way to re-election. There are dangerous trends toward withdrawing funding from environmental protection, which is also our protection. Your firm voice in opposition to this will make a difference; so will your support of progressive measures.

Every being on the planet is ultimately dependent on photosynthesis, the process by which plants use energy from light to synthesize carbohydrates from carbon dioxide and water, producing food and releasing oxygen into the atmosphere.

PHOTOSYNTHESIS

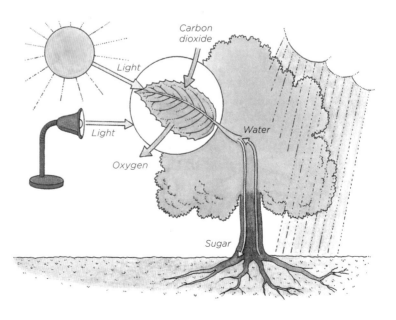

Carbon dioxide

Light

Light

Oxygen

Water

Sugar

HOW TO CHOOSE A THERAPIST

The emphasis in this book is on helping you to use the great variety of approaches to health and healing that are becoming increasingly available to all of us in our homes. As you will have noted, many of these approaches require that you first establish contact with a therapist or teacher who can explain and demonstrate the fine points, without which the therapy simply will not be effective.

Once this vital information has been passed on to you, you will be able to carry on without difficulty on your own. But it can be difficult to take this first step, so I thought a few practical tips would be in order.

The best answer is a recommendation from a friend or someone else you trust to give good advice. It will be especially helpful if the person to whom you turn has had personal experience on which to base the recommendations. However, if help does not come in this way, what can you do then? One of several different routes may be open to you.

Go to your doctor's office or health center and ask for advice. They may or may not be sympathetic to such a request, but you may be pleasantly surprised. The right person may help at the clinic, or their database may contain the name of a person to whom they regularly refer patients.

Search the internet for information sources in your local area. Seek out a natural health center in your area. Even if the right teacher or therapist is not on the scene, they may be able to direct you to that person. Natural practitioners tend to form a network of information that can turn into a network of referral when needed.

Your nearest health food store is often a good source of such information, since complementary/alternative therapists often use or recommend their products and leave their names there for referral purposes. Therapists may also have their details listed in the Yellow Pages and local newspapers, as well as at citizen advice and information centers and libraries.

If these local efforts fail, the next step is to contact a national organization that maintains a listing of therapists and teachers in all parts of the country. There may or may not be a charge for the information. Most organizations will gladly give you information about themselves, so that you can see if they are well-established, how many members they represent, and other things of interest, such as whether they have a code of ethics. You may also be able to find out about the qualifications of people who are listed as members of organizations.

The final decision is yours. Once you have done all the checking you want to do, all that remains is to meet the teacher or therapist who will instruct you in person. You will be able to sense whether the person is clearly in command of the professed subject, and whether that person just as clearly has your interests at heart.

You should be ready and willing to pass on a recommendation to others, based on your own experience as you go through the process of acquiring information about self-administered therapy. You may have been helped in this way yourself, so why not help someone else.

INDEX

Italic entries refer to illustrations

CREDITS

We would like to thank and acknowledge the following for supplying images reproduced in this book:

Key: l (left), r (right), a (above), b (below), c (center)

www.shutterstock.com: Pensiri (leaf illustrations used throughout); pp.1, 46 Cozine; pp.2al, 33 natalia bulatova; pp.2cl, 200 coka; pp.2bl, 172–173 Antonova Ganna; pp.2r, 153 Wassana Panapute; pp.4, 83 NaturalBox; pp.5l, 247 Larisa Lofitskaya; pp.5r, 106 Milenie; p.6l Eskymaks; p.6r, 65 ifong; pp.7l, 109, 139 HelloRF Zcool; pp.7r, 189a Leonardo da; pp.8, 233 Olga Miltsova; pp.10, 187 Y Photo Studio; pp.11, 145 Marilyn barbone; pp.12–13 Yellowj; pp.14, 31, 37a, 73, 78, 135, 185, 195, 224 Africa Studio; p.15al New Africa; p.15ar Panida_Noi; p.15bc Passakom sakulphan; p.16 RobSimonART; p.17b Floral Deco; p.18 Orawan Pattarawimonchai; pp.19, 63, 103 javi_indy; p.20 Ileish Anna; pp.21, 147 Daxiao Productions; p.22 Seasontime; p.24 M. Unal Ozmen; p.25 Marina Bakush; p.26b Manfred Ruckszio; p.29 puhhha; p.30 beta7; p.35 mimagephotography; pp.37b, 238–239 Evgeny Karandaev; pp.39, 107, 144 Antonina Vlasova; p.41 Nataly Studio; pp.43, 191 Microgen; p.44 Rimma Bondarenko; p.45 Poznyakov; p.47br Valentyn Volkov; pp.48, 60 Dionisvera; p.49 Cultura Motion; p.50 Shebeko; p.51 Gts; pp.53, 127 Stock-Asso; p.54 Artem Furman; p.57 Maren Winter; p.58 Wayhome studio; p.61 Abo Photography; p.64 Craevschii Family; p.66 areeya_ann; p.69 Tatevosian Yana; p.71 Jacek Chabraszewski; p.74 Bjoern Wylezich; p.76 Fereshteh; p.81 Tatiana Volgutova; p.84 Kung Min Ju; p.86 donfiore; p.89 Lukiyanova Natalia frenta; p.90 saltodemata; p.91b vainillaychile; p.92 Blackday; p.95 Kinga; p.96, 237 iva; p.99 Oleksandr Nagaiets; p.100a Vladislav Noseek; p.101 Melodia plus photos; p.108 Alexander Raths; p.111 Max Topchii; p.112 Syda Productions; p.114 margouillat photo; p.116 AVprophoto;

p.117 Dragon Images; p.118 Pattakorn Uttarasak; pp.119, 193 Lucky Business; p.121a LMproduction; p.123 Viktor Gladkov; p.124 Shustikova Inessa; p.125 Ludmilla Ivashchenko; p.128 iordani; p.131 Odua Images; p.132 Diana Taliun; p.136b SiNeeKan; p.140 vitals; p.143 lev radin; p.147 Daxiao Productions; p.148 Korke; p.149bl Business-Creations; p.151a peterzsuzsa; p.154 Alena Ozerova; p.155b romantitov; p.156 Pixel Embargo; p.157 Marina Sliusarenko; p.158 Swapan Photography; p.159 DR Travel Photo and Video; p.161 S_L; p.163 Zdenka Darula; p.164 Albina Glisic; p.167 Andrew Mayovskyy; p.168 Jack Hong; pp.171, 217 Monkey Business Images; p.175 Serg64; p.176 bigacis; p.177 baibaz; p.178 Ariwasabi; p.181 nd3000; p.182 ESB Professional; p.184 Val Thoermer; p.201b Tyler Olson; p.202 Sebastian Kaulitzki; pp.205, 206l, 222 fizkes; p.206r Robert Kneschke; p.208 suns07butterfly; p.209 Natalia Hirshfeld; p.210 May_Chanikran; p.212 wavebreakmedia; p.213 Africa Rising; p.215 Marina Demidova; p.219 karamysh; p.221 Antonio Guillem; p.223 Photographee.eu; p.225 Paul Vinten; p.226 Potapov Alexander (cl), Summer Photographer (cr), Mykola Mazuryk (r); p.227 parsobchai Ngammoa (l), Luis Echeverri Urrea (cl), bergamont (cr), Piotr_pabijan (r); p.228 Monika Wisniewska; p.229 Leszek Glasner; p.231 Olena Yakobchuk; p.232 Jason Squyres; pp.234–235 Anna Ok; p.236 TunedIn by Westend61; p.240 SasaStock; p.241 Patricia Chumillas; pp.242–243 Chamille White; p.244 Dima Sobko; p.245 Gilles Lougassi; p.246 YKKStudio.

www.StockFood.co.uk: p.105 Reschke, Mandy.

All other photographs and illustrations are the copyright of Quarto Publishing plc. While every effort has been made to credit contributors, Quarto would like to apologize should there have been any omissions or errors—and would be pleased to make the appropriate correction for future editions of the book.

AUTHOR'S ACKNOWLEDGEMENTS

I wish to offer my heartfelt thanks to: my wife Bets, who has given me every kind of loving support and encouragement during the seemingly endless process of writing this book, and for her specific contributions in the areas of nutrition and reflexology; Michelle Pickering, my lifeline at Quarto Publishing, whose patient and intelligent guidance has been a blessing; the other staff at Quarto—artists, designers, photographers, and all—whose excellent work contributes so mightily to making this book what it is.

The principal sources for the recommended levels of nutritional supplements on page 179 are: Andrew Weil, M.D.—Harvard Medical School graduate, faculty member of University of Arizona College of Medicine, founder of the Center of Integrative Medicine, Tucson, Arizona, author, and lecturer; Alan Gaby, M.D.—author and lecturer in nutritional medicine and past president of American Holistic Medication of Association; Jeffrey Bland, Ph.D.—nutritional biochemist, author, and lecturer.

Note: This book was previously published in 1997 as *The Complete Book of Complementary Therapies* by Peter Albright, M.D. Additional text (First Aid for Pain, pp.14–18) has been contributed by Richard Thomas from his book *The Complete Book of Natural Pain Relief*.